Notes on Yoga

Notes on Yoga
The Legacy of Vanda Scaravelli

Diane Long
and Sophy Hoare

YOGAWORDS

Notes on Yoga: The Legacy of Vanda Scaravelli

First published by YogaWords, an imprint of Pinter & Martin Ltd 2016

© 2016 Diane Long and Sophy Hoare

ISBN 978-1-906756-45-1
Also available as ebook

British Library Cataloguing-in-Publication Data
A catalogue record for this book is available from the British Library.

Set in Gill Sans and Optima

Printed and bound in the EU by Hussar Books

This book has been printed on paper that is sourced and harvested from sustainable forests and is FSC accredited.

Pinter & Martin Ltd
6 Effra Parade
London SW2 1PS

Notes on Yoga was edited and designed by Annette Heyer and Lise Bratton.

Cover designed by Annette Heyer, Lise Bratton and Rupert Wilks at Annette's Walmer Crescent Studio, Glasgow.

For Vanda, the guiding light shining throughout this book

Contents

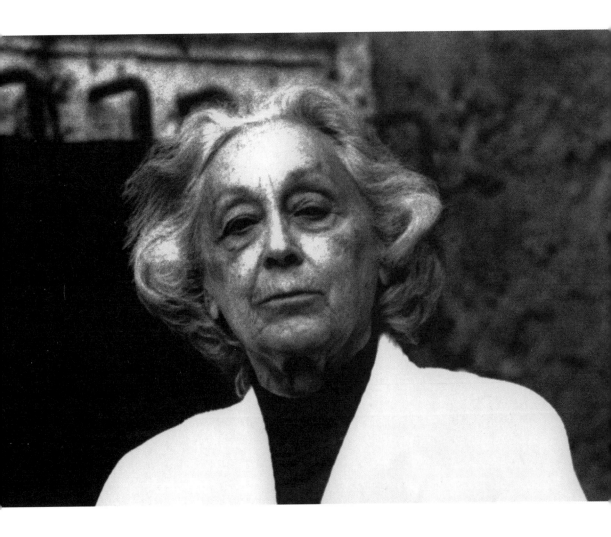

'Is it possible to have a different attitude in which a new intelligence, not imposed by authority but born from interest, attention and sensitivity, will emerge and in which body and mind, fused in one single action, are collaborating together? It is just this revolutionary attitude that we are going to discover through a new discipline in the practice of yoga.'

Vanda Scaravelli[1]

About this Book

Vanda Scaravelli developed an approach to yoga that is radically different from most forms of yoga taught today. Her practice evolved over a period of forty years, during which time she accepted a small number of individual students, all of whom were teachers.

Diane Long was the first of her regular students and studied with her for twenty-three years. Sophy Hoare met Vanda during the period when she was writing *Awakening the Spine*, and worked with her intensively once or twice a year from then on.

Since the publication of her book, this form of yoga has spread throughout the world and Vanda Scaravelli is now well known.

The nature of the practice is subtle and, therefore, difficult to grasp. Vanda's book inspires through its philosophy and images, but it does not go into detail when describing the practice of asanas. The teaching can be easily misinterpreted. Her approach to yoga was more revolutionary than many people realise, even those who attend 'Scaravelli' classes.

In *Notes on Yoga: The Legacy of Vanda Scaravelli*, we have responded to requests from our students for a book that would help them with their practice. The result is this handbook, which consists of both suggestions and personal accounts of the experience of being taught by Vanda.

The structure of the book invites the reader to refer to different aspects of the text at different times. The photographs show playing at asanas and exploring within asanas. They depict sequences of movements through the body, not the held and accomplished poses.

Our approach throughout this book, as in our teaching, is to help students to let go of old assumptions about yoga. We are not attempting to explain how to do the yoga asanas; instead, we explore the asanas from a different perspective.

In ancient Indian philosophy, the ultimate, impersonal reality of the universe, Brahman, could be apprehended only by understanding what is not Brahman. This form of enquiry was known as 'neti, neti' (literally 'not this, not this'.) This yoga practice cannot be clearly prescribed or delineated, because the attempt to do so takes us further away from understanding. There is always more to discover than we already know.

When Vanda was teaching, she used a mixture of Sanskrit and English words for the asanas and, for the sake of ease and clarity, we are doing the same here. For example, we refer to Shoulder-stand rather than Salamba Sarvangasana, and Dog Pose rather than Urdhva Mukha Svanasana. But we refer to Virasana and Uttanasana because they are easy to say and widely used. Throughout, 'asana', 'pose' and 'posture' are interchangeable.

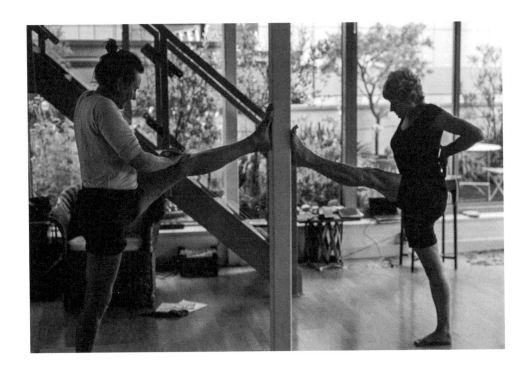

About Us

Sophy

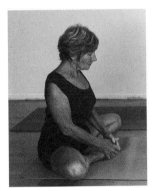

When I worked with Vanda, I stayed in her house for a week or ten days at a time. Every morning she would summon me at about eleven o'clock, when she had finished her own practice. Sometimes I had a lesson on my own and, sometimes, one of her weekly students would join us. When I was on my own, the practice was always intense and we worked hard and long. When other students were present it was instructive to watch how Vanda helped them with their practice. I noticed that she tended to go with their natural inclination; if they wanted to go slowly and take rests, she let them go at their own pace; if they had a more active rhythm, she would encourage it; if they wanted to focus on sitting and breathing, she readily acquiesced. This was in contrast to the teachers I had known at home who tried to 'wake up' 'lazy' students with vigorous poses, or calm down 'restless' students with quieter ones. I began to understand the meaning of going with the body and not against it.

After a few years I met Diane at Vanda's house and we shared some lessons. I had met her briefly once or twice in London and I was immediately struck by the change in her body since I had last seen her. I recognised the same quality of movement that Vanda had been demonstrating to me. This was the first time I had seen it so clearly in another person, and I was fascinated by it. If it was there in two people, then it must be possible for me to find it! Vanda was already eighty-three when I met her and every time I left her, I wondered if I would see her again. Since this practice turned out to be what my body had always been seeking, I asked Diane whether she would teach me and my students. That was the beginning of a long and fruitful collaboration. Because the practice constantly reveals surprises, I had the impression that Vanda, and Diane, could always surprise me. There has never been a moment of dullness. From our first meeting, I have continued to learn from Diane and I am honoured to have helped her write this book.

What appeals to me most about this approach to yoga is that it gives me the key to unlock my body and become freer than I have been before. There is a feeling of boundlessness and aliveness, calm energy that comes instantaneously. I recognise it as clean and true and 'right'. It cuts through all personal preoccupations. I love its simplicity and its complexity, the fact that it can go on deepening and enriching itself for as long as I live. I love the fact that there are no rules, no authority outside the practice itself. I like the paradoxes contained within it and the poetic and philosophical reflections it can give rise to, if I have a mind to follow. And I like the fact that it is counter-cultural and questions our habits and assumptions, individually and collectively.

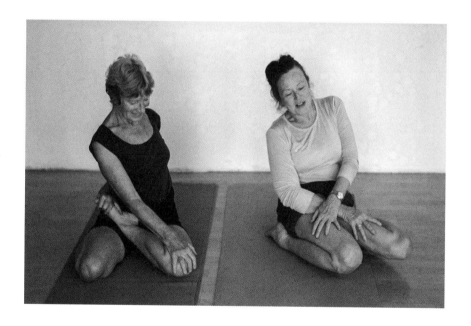

Diane

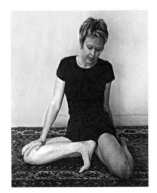

Sophy is vital to the writing of this book. When she invited me to London, I had great enthusiasm and love for what I was doing, but I was probably unintelligible to most students. My body was awakened by Vanda's persistence and wisdom, but my words did not have the same confidence as my body language. I remember more than a few of Sophy's students turning to her with puzzled looks; she would help by saying, 'What I think she means is....'

Before meeting Vanda my study of yoga was didactic — it had become a growing compendium of information, which imprisoned my body. In the process of unlearning, my body and mind resonated with Vanda's teaching. She used few words and, after my previous experience, this was a relief.

Sophy and I shared the conviction that the body could be transformed with this approach, and the results were deep and surprising. Bodies changed shape and were awakened to an inner listening. We began to teach together occasionally; Sophy was more verbal, while I was more dependent on the visual.

Students began asking for a book, so I went away on a retreat with my notes and scribbles, writing down what I could. On reading it through, I realised it was all about Vanda and was not going to help others with their practice. I was not writing from my own convictions and understanding.

Even though students spoke of the differences in how Sophy and I taught, I became convinced that there should be more than a single voice behind this endeavour; together we could bring forth something more interesting. Her skills as a writer have given me courage in the process of creating this small book and my words have gained more clarity. Equally, Sophy now has more trust in the wordless music of her body. I am grateful for her participation.

The yoga Vanda introduced me to has enabled me to discover deep and harmonious connections within the body. These pathways invite play with the asanas — going with, through, beyond them. So much is revealed, and I am left feeling refreshed and alert. It is a practice which, sometimes directly, sometimes indirectly, sometimes by chance, reveals magical connections between lightness and rest.

At times the breath appears to unfold a movement and at other times movement appears to unfold as breath. Each day this practice amazes and surprises me, allowing me to listen more alertly to the profound intelligence of the body.

Becoming a Beginner

*'There are two ways to live. You can live as if nothing is a miracle,
or you can live as if everything is a miracle.'*

attributed to Albert Einstein

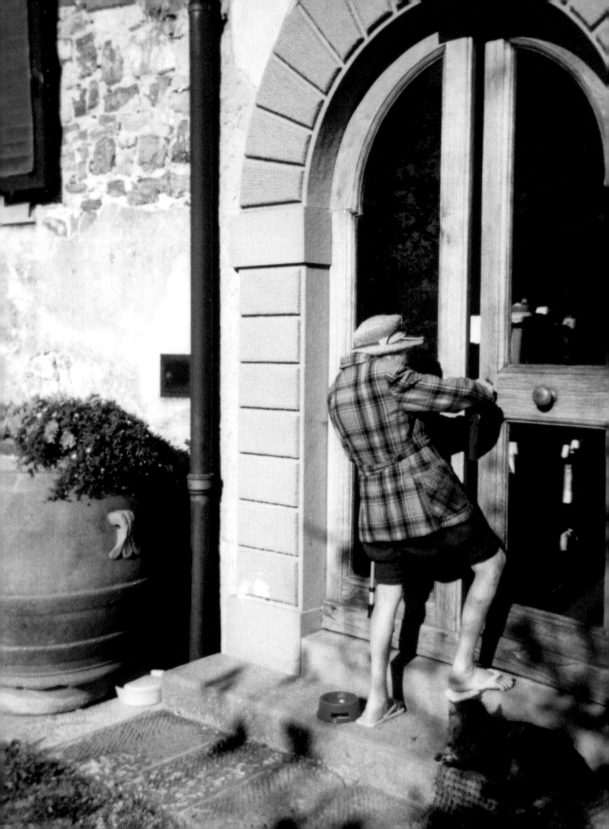

Meeting Vanda

Diane

One day, at a Tai Chi demonstration in Florence, a tiny woman in the crowd beckoned to me. She told me her name was Vanda and invited me to visit her at her home near Florence. I was intrigued, but so busy that, after several months, I still hadn't followed up her invitation. Then a friend invited me for lunch at the home of an Italian signora, an acquaintance of his mother. He explained to me that she was an eccentric Roman countess who had recently moved to one of her family villas in Fiesole.

The door opened and there was the same Vanda who had told me to visit her, taking my wrist and leading me away from my friend. When she dropped my wrist, I found myself in a small room with a grand piano, a large mirror and a brilliant pomegranate tree outside double glass doors.

'Watch,' I was told as she began a series of Backbends, more beautifully and gracefully than I had ever seen. 'What is your name? Ah, Diana. Watch, Diana, do you see?'

'Now,' as she finally stopped, with a twinkling look in her eye, 'I want you to study with me — and do not tell anyone.'

Working with Vanda was completely different from what I had been doing before. Suddenly my accomplishment in asana meant nothing. 'What is your hurry? Why don't you relax?' Yet, she was asking me to work harder than I had ever done. Her instructions were simple. I would be abruptly brought back to begin anew, to understand more precisely what she was asking of me. It took repeated efforts before she was satisfied. I realised that a different and difficult journey had begun.

This new approach to learning stopped me from moving too quickly. I observed Vanda's movements closely. How did she engage the rest of her body when one movement was made? There seemed to be total involvement, her body was relaxed and connected. It seemed impossible to acquire the grace that I saw in her, but I was captivated by what I saw and there was no turning back.

Soon, I was having lessons three, four, five times a week, however difficult that was to arrange. Then, somehow, a little at a time, my body began to respond. Vanda seemed to have the key to unlocking my body; she was teaching me how to listen. Trying to imitate her movements, I began to perceive my body differently. I had become accustomed to immediate results, but now I began to trust the process she was introducing me to.

I began thinking of the teachers I had had in the past. Were they trying to help students to become more intelligent with themselves? I remember being told by each 'senior' teacher that what I was doing was wrong. Yet, it was simply what the previous teacher had told me to do! There seemed to be no consensus — how confusing it all became! The very first time I worked with Vanda, I sensed the deep connection between her own practice and what she was teaching. She taught with clarity and integrity, demanding these qualities from her students. I learned from her how yoga can help us to rediscover the poetry we carry within our bodies.

The elegance of Vanda's movements seemed to be based on an economy of effort. 'Do not push. Do not pull,' she said again and again. It takes time to acquire the ability to use less effort as new networks of muscles develop that displace the habitual ones. The lungs become an extra pair of arms. The spine receives the weight of the arms and then releases it. The spine receives the weight of the legs and releases it. Hands and feet gain more freedom of movement and definition, and a feeling of lightness pervades the body. Muscles do not need to be over-stretched, nor joints inhibited in their movements.

I did not realise that what I saw in Vanda's movements, I already possessed; we all already possess this wisdom. Watching my teacher's body helped me begin to make friends with my own. Vanda was always learning from herself, even as she taught. She helped me believe in the changes that lead to new beginnings and showed what fun we could have allowing them to happen.

For many years I accompanied yoga students and teachers to their first lessons with Vanda. How often I watched them become frustrated, unsure of what had happened, unable to start all over again. Sometimes, they were in tears as they realised the enormity of the change that was being made available to them, and they did not yet perceive how delightful the journey could be.

During one of my very first lessons with Vanda, she asked me how much I practised. How proudly I replied, 'Two hours in the morning and two hours in *the afternoon.'* She smiled, *'Noooo — too much. Do not take yourself so seriously,'* and there was a warm, deep laugh, wonderfully contagious. How much more playful the learning of yoga could become.

If we can see ourselves as slightly ridiculous, it is easier to meet the marvels of what the body might reveal — unburdening not only the asanas, but also ourselves. Playfulness brings innocence, the opposite of what I thought it meant to be a 'good yoga teacher'. We can learn to orchestrate our own practice. The best teachers are pleased by this.

If we give our attention to working well — just the right amount, no more — an undoing takes place and we experience repose and renewal. After a lesson with Vanda, I would be told, *'Finished, rest.'* I would lie down, she would sit behind my head and take my skull in her hands, lean back and draw it away from my spine. My body obeyed a bit at a time; there was surrender, and yet more release took place. She would then massage my forehead, covering my eyes with a rice bag. I rested, and was refreshed and hungry — lunch was ready.

Sophy

My relationship with Vanda started with a phone call. My former teacher rang me to ask whether I would like to have a lesson with Vanda while she was in London. Suddenly Vanda was talking to me. *'Come,'* she said to me. *'Come,'* and put the phone down abruptly.

During this first lesson, Vanda asked me why I had not been to see her in Florence. Taken aback, I started to explain that I had a busy life with a husband and four children, whereupon she told me that I should visit her as soon as possible, and to bring all my children with me if I wished.

From that time on, I visited Vanda (without the children) once or twice a year. After a week of lessons I would fly back to London, almost intoxicated with well-being and enthusiasm and, on arriving home, was confronted with the problem of my own practice; even more worryingly, what was I going to teach my students? I was being asked to let go of my former practice completely. The new could not be grafted on to the old, and I began to realise that the two could not be merged; that the new, in its wholeness, was uncompromising.

This appealed to me in theory, but how was I to find it? My visits to Italy were few. In the meantime, I was on my own, floundering around, trying to recall what I had done with Vanda, trying to reproduce in my body what she had brought about — as if by magic. After more than twenty years' experience of yoga and fifteen years of teaching, I was a beginner again. I knew nothing. But I kept searching and trying, and explained to my students that I was learning to do yoga in a completely different way. Miraculously, most of them trusted what I was doing and stayed with me.

Because I stayed in Vanda's house, I had plenty of opportunity to observe the way she moved. Although she was in her eighties, she rarely allowed me to help her with fetching and carrying. I was impressed by the slow, roundabout, confident way in which she reached for things from high shelves, or carried heavy bags of shopping, or simply walked along the road. Sometimes, she reminded me of a cat stabbing at something with its paw, or a bird ruffling its wings. She always looked for the easiest way — the *'most beautiful'* way as she would call it.

I talked to Diane about this practice and invited her to come to London to teach me and my students; this was the beginning of our collaboration. Now I had another teacher whom I could see two or even three times a year — but still, I was on my own in between, and I missed being able to go to a regular class. What's more, rather than finding that Diane could explain the practice to me in clear and simple terms as I had hoped, almost the opposite occurred. She used little explanation and even threw me into greater confusion by telling me to do the opposite of what Vanda had said to me! Eventually, I realised that what Vanda often said was a description of what happens when the body pulls together as a whole — finally, after years of practice. I began to learn from Diane that many other changes need to happen in the body before Vanda's descriptions become a reality.

Perhaps I would have progressed more quickly if I had been able to work with my teachers every week. Perhaps I wouldn't have struggled with my own practice so much. But, if we have regular, if infrequent, access to a teacher we trust, then the process will inevitably unfold. Now that there are more teachers of this approach to yoga, most students don't have to wait for months between lessons, and practice at home can be better supported than it was for me.

Developing Trust

This new beginning can be disorienting; a good teacher guides us through the unfamiliar territory, and the pathways of the body begin to reveal themselves. Old habits are changed.

Be careful when choosing your teacher. Sometimes teachers speak from a shallow well of understanding. Academic knowledge and paper qualifications are not important. Beware of those who impose rules and permit no questions.

Even when you have found an inspiring teacher, experiment with the information you are given. It is up to you, the student, to bring an enquiring mind.

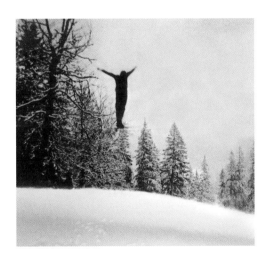

'The mind that is not baffled is not employed.
The impeded stream is the one that sings.'

Wendell Berry[2]

Establishing a Practice

One of the most common habits, which may prevent us from making progress, is trying too hard. The desire to understand and to effect change can cause us to use willpower and force. This fragments our movements and a vicious circle is set up — we feel that we are failing to 'get it', which prompts more misguided effort and leads to tension. If we accept that the process takes time, that it is necessary to not know, then we can let go of unhelpful habits and see what is revealed. We are entering a process that unfolds gradually.

We have to question how we use our bodies, in every way. Sites of resistance and pain most often result from lack of integration. It is important to recognise tension: shoulders, neck, jaws, knees, inner groins, buttocks, thighs, calves, feet, hands. We can dilute tension simply by noticing where a part of the body is not enjoying its range of motion, its ability to make more than one use of itself.

A tense, dull body can misinterpret the information we give to it, which may cause fragmentation, confusion, pain or injury. The well-ordered and harmonious body is our study. There develops a resonance between how we feel and how the body works. Talk to your body. Listen to your body.

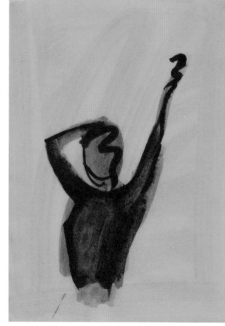

Become lighter and see what that suggests. Investigate the structure of your feet, the structure of your hands. Investigate the connections between the large joints of the body and soften the larger outer muscles to feel what is happening beneath them. Use your eyes and your imagination. Be playful; take a scientific attitude, becoming curious and questioning assumptions.

A good teacher can help you become more creative in your practice. Make friends with your body!

Some Suggestions

A short practice every day is more effective than occasional long sessions. It is the attention given that is most important.

You do not need a special yoga place. You can make any space special.

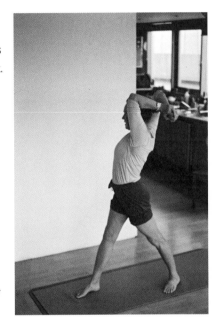

Though there are many asanas, most are variations of simple positions, such as standing, sitting, lying down, upside down, bending backwards, with a twist here and there.

Notice the quality of your breath, before, during and after your practice. Do not try to control it.

The practice is about exploration, not performance. Asanas are not goals but frameworks for finding connections within the body.

Don't try to remember everything from the class — one or two things can be plenty to feed your practice.

Let go of the concept of achievement and doing. Try not to anticipate your next move.

Practise when your energy is best.

Some Misconceptions

Yoga does not have to be adapted for different situations — yoga for pregnancy, yoga for children, yoga for slimmers, yoga for the over-50s, yoga for runners, etc. It is unnecessary and even confusing. Yoga should bring us to a clearer understanding of the body and breath which can only be therapeutic, whatever limitations one may have. If we give our attention to the body's connections and to integration, our attention is distracted from our injuries and healing often occurs. Our own deepening practice should enable us to teach anyone.

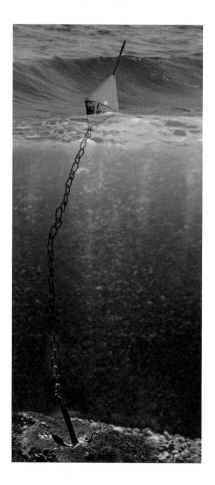

Grounding

Sometimes being 'grounded' is mistaken for heaviness. While working with Vanda, we were often wonderstruck by the lightness in her body. She seemed to defy gravity. This perplexed us because of the emphasis she placed on *'Down! Down!'* Later we realised that lightness is never sacrificed.

Most of us are too heavy on the ground; we have dropped our arches and our centre of gravity, have lost our spring.

Taking the burden of weight away from the legs and feet brings the centre of gravity upwards to lighten the upper part of the body, including shoulders and arms.

The body is built to work most efficiently when the centre of gravity is lifted. Then, we are able to connect with the ground through our deep roots, engaging our heels and knees, without compromising lightness.

Pulling the shoulders down

Many of us have, at some time, been told to pull our shoulders away from our ears. Pulling the shoulders down compromises the integrity of the spine. The shoulder girdle is not meant to be fixed.

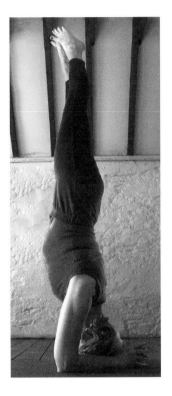

'We should associate the shoulder girdle, in our imagination, more closely with the head than with the chest, if we are to centre the upper weights successfully on the spine. This converts a side-load into the more easily balanced top-load. In the primary patterns of movement, the thorax and pelvis work together, with breathing rhythms adjusted to the coordinated whole, while shoulders and arms follow the dictates of the head.'

Mabel Todd[3]

Tucking the tail-bone under

Tucking the tail-bone under, eg in Dog Pose or Backbend, fixes the pelvis which, like the shoulder girdle, should be free. The pelvis is a responsive, mobile shock-absorber between the legs and the spine.

Holding postures

Holding still makes hundreds of muscles overwork. It brings on fatigue and prevents us from finding the 'inner dance' that Vanda referred to.

There is no such thing as a final or completed position. Through the vehicle of the asana, using the natural rhythm of the breath, we refine the way we inhabit the body.

Strengthening the abdominal muscles

Forcefully engaging the abdominal muscles prevents access to deeper muscles in the pelvis and along the lower spine. Do not let the abdominal muscles become a restricting corset.

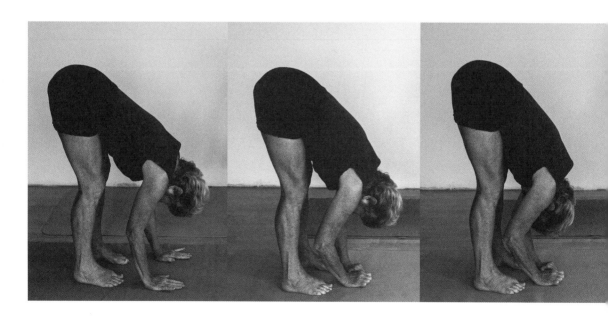

Stretching

When exploring asanas on your own, do not deliberately stretch. The concept of stretching is superficial and linear.

Muscles release from their centre outwards, giving more freedom and mobility to their attached joints. Use your imagination; it will lead you to discover real physical connections which are waiting to be restored. Forbid yourself to push or brace with your hands, arms, feet and legs. Find out whether there is another way.

Keep your breathing relaxed and light. Don't try to synchronise your movements with the breath, but rather let the breath respond naturally; if you are attentive, the breath will deepen.

We can find ways of approaching the hidden layers of the body — the spine and its muscles, the inside of the joints, the inside of the ribs, and even the lungs. We can't fly there instantly. We undo the obstacles a little at a time.

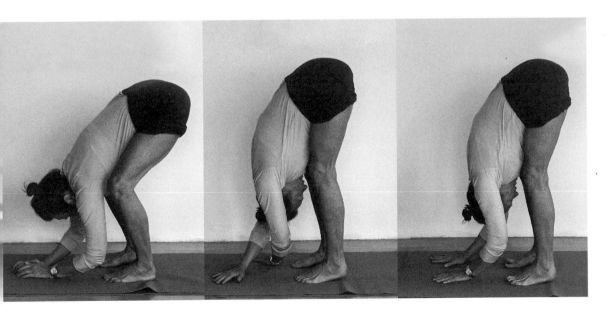

The Quality of Practice

*'The same stream of life that runs through my veins night and day
runs through the world and dances in rhythmic measures.'*

Rabindranath Tagore[4]

p cedatur. Siqs inuec̃ui est p cedatur. Siqs pcegrenus est p cedatur.

Siqs æthenus est p cedatur. Cuiz cutez non est p cedatur. Iatz beneđ.

Explecto barpensmo. Cuietur̃·

fiehtr ad fonct · cetñ ã · hãc· Domine pctegenos· dñe gu

bnacnos· Emmanuhel nob cuzdtur ædluucenos· keyne ley

son. Xp̃e leyson· keyne leyson. Xp̃e audinos· Sce marhce otcep

nobis· xp̃e audinos· Sce michahel otce pnobis xp̃e audinos· Alii

fceccecñz leĉ· Rp̃ gñ cib; ccensndo inchoso· Rẽ micecncur· qñ

λ xxxxiiii

jep̃· ad ala ccte· cetñ ã · hãc·

Iaso sct· Rluxcecr um etũ sepcnso cuce p̃useu· Repostce pgecur sce· ut·

Tteencruum; pigne sceequce· Doxce scupscuhs cche o· keepigis

keyn iii· Al leluice· Al lelu ice· Al leluice· Gloñ ce in excel

su de o· Blucefter pccx· Al leluice· Al lelu ice· Al leluice·

Music

'Musical training is a more potent instrument than any other because
rhythm and harmony find their way into the inward places of the soul.'
Plato[5]

Vanda was a classical pianist and spent many years exploring how to play
without tension. With the same attitude, she looked for a harmonious
way of doing yoga.

Diane

Towards the end of Vanda's life, I would arrive early for my lesson, sit on the
step outside her room and listen to her playing the piano. Often she would play
a sequence of notes over and over again, until she seemed pleased with the sound.
Afterwards, she would add a beginning and an end to the sequence, playing the
whole piece only once. Then I would knock on her window.

Musical terms illuminate our practice. Work becomes play. Rhythm, rest, pause,
movement, timing, piano, andante — these words can apply to yoga. Vanda used
the expression 'tuning the body' to describe how we start exploring a posture.

In yoga, we develop a subtle control that does not disturb the body's
equilibrium. We have to re-learn this in each practice, inviting internal muscles
to come alive. Just as a cat moves when stalking a mouse, when we place any
part of the body on the ground, we do so without heaviness attached to it.

Before meeting Vanda, both of us were taught yoga in a way that was prescriptive
and analytical; exploration was not encouraged. Vanda gave simple instructions that
were repeated over and over until she was pleased with our response. This forced
us to wake up to the interpretive quality of what we were doing.

There is a similarity with chanting, in which resonance and listening become more acute. The body acts and the mind responds, each listening to the other.

We can become aware of the too little, too much, too strong, too weak. There can be intensity in simple asanas and ease in complicated ones. We develop skill by moving in unusual ways; even taking detours. We notice the difference between one side of the body and the other. The musical quality reveals itself as having other dimensions — 'on the way to', 'going through', 'around and out from'.

Vanda spoke often of the expansion that comes in the middle of the wave-like movement in asana. During and after a movement we wait, briefly, assessing how it feels. Often the body responds spontaneously, surprising us, waking us up to a more alert state of rest. Whatever the pace, the quality of rest must be present.

Like the instruments in an orchestra, the parts of the body continue to be involved after we have invited them in, even when we have diverted our attention elsewhere. What has already been done is not lost.

Music can link us to an ancient part of ourselves. It is often used as therapy to regain speech after strokes.

The neurologist Oliver Sacks relates his experience of the healing effects of music in his book, *A Leg to Stand On*, in which he charts the stages of his recovery from a severe leg injury. While struggling alone down a mountainside with his leg broken and useless, he was tempted to give up and die, but a voice willed him not to. He writes: *'There came to my aid now melody, rhythm and music (what Kant calls the "quickening art"). Before […] I had muscled myself along, moving by main force with my very strong arms. Now […] I was musicked along. I did not contrive this. It happened to me. I fell into a rhythm, guided by a sort of marching or rowing song […].'*

Weeks later, in hospital, Sacks described his fear of learning to walk again. His leg did not seem to belong to him; it felt alien and useless. *'And suddenly — into the silence […] came music […]. And, as suddenly, in the moment that this inner music started […] and in the very moment that my motor music, my kinetic melody, my walking, came back — in this self-same moment **the leg came back**. Suddenly, […] with no transition whatever, the leg felt alive, and real, and mine […].'*

Music helped him to walk without thinking how to do it. As Sacks says, *'What is required is a sort of "trick". […] The alienated part […] is "deceived" into action'.*

This is the way in which we can work with yoga, allowing parts of the body to be spontaneously drawn into the whole.

'Every disease is a musical problem, every cure a musical solution.'

Novalis[6]

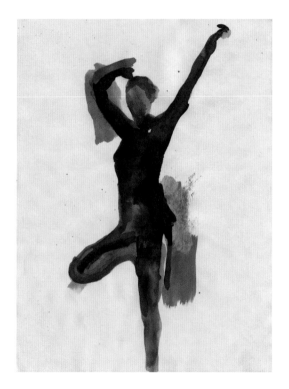

Rhythm is a part of our lives from before we are born. When we begin exploring our relationship with gravity, powerful internal rhythms can be felt.

We counteract gravity, working against it to use its strength. In this way, we 'open out from' and 'grow up through' the centre of our spine.

When we are relaxed, we can observe that the resting phase of the heart is longer than its beat and the exhalation is longer than the inhalation. When the spine comes alive, the quality of the breath is improved — becoming easier, lighter, freer. The spine, the lungs and the internal 'core' muscles are inextricably linked.

'You know that our lungs lie around the heart, so the air passing through them envelops the heart. Having collected your mind with you, lead it into the channel of breathing through which air reaches the heart and, together with this inhaled air, force your mind to descend into the heart and to remain there — the mind, when it unites with the heart, is filled with unspeakable joy and delight.'

Nicephorus[7]

Language

anguage is a tool by which we perceive as well as a means of communication. How we use language in relating to our body, affects how we perceive our body.

When we start to learn yoga, we can be confused by unfamiliar patterns and connections. If we do not resist the confusion, we can create islands of clarity and understanding and, little by little, these join up. Our world opens into a delightful new dimension.

Spoken language is a powerful tool for learning the body's language. When we are changing ingrained habits, we can speak instructions to ourselves, silently or aloud. Enriching the words we use

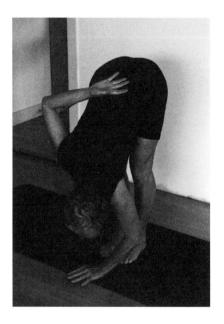

triggers a clearer response. Why tell the body the same things in the same ways? Rather than saying, 'stretch, push, pull, hold, bend, extend,' find words which are more enticing: 'arrange, rearrange, cultivate, connect, invite, gather, release, allow, receive, enjoy, expand.'

It is important to wait between actions to allow the body's intelligence to lead you. When a response comes, hold it lightly and the next response will be clearer. You will begin to recognise structural and internal connections, and discover the body's poetic quality.

When a new connection is found, we have an urge to define it. It is best to hold lightly to these definitions. The body reveals its intelligence at deeper and deeper levels; we need to be freshly present to listen. We nearly always recognise what is right. The new sensation may trigger a distant memory, the impression of 'coming home'. This is confirmation.

It is harder to recognise what is wrong, ie, fragmented. Our habits blind us and, at first, our practice can be frustrating. It is important to have a teacher who can help you find your way, through language, demonstration and hands-on adjustments. We become aware of the connections that exist between the senses of hearing, touch and sight. This strengthens our proprioceptive intelligence, sometimes referred to as our sixth sense.

Imaginative instructions help us to elicit precise well-ordered connections within the body, yet sometimes, an image is enough in itself. The image of the eagle with outstretched wings and legs extended downwards, shown repeatedly by Vanda to her students, was more vivid than words.

Keep in mind that words are clues, hints, indications; they cannot give an exact representation of what is happening inside the body. It is up to us to interpret, to find out what really lies behind the words. We are faced again and again with the apparent contradiction between the possibilities of the imagination and the precision of the body's elegant architecture. In the process of refining our practice, what we find is always a surprise; none of our habits or previous knowledge will take us directly there. It is as if it has come out of the blue, like a gift, in response to our attentiveness and our willingness not to know.

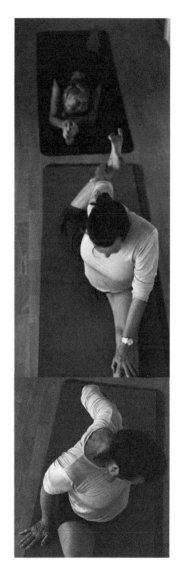

'The walnut tree
One day it will see God
And so, to be sure,
It develops its being in roundness
And holds out ripe arms to him.'
                                    Rainer Maria Rilke[8]

The Brain

> 'The cerebral cortex does not simply learn, it is always learning how to learn. It can reorganise itself.'
>
> Michael M. Merzenich[9]

The most outstanding feature of the brain is its malleability, reflected in the innumerable potential combinations of its cells. According to Mark Solms and Oliver Turnbull in their book, *The Brain and the Inner World*, *'the fine organisation of the brain is literally sculpted by the environment in which it finds itself — far more so than any other organ in the body, and over much longer periods of time.'*[10]

When practising yoga, we use the pre-frontal lobes of the brain, which enable us to imagine actions in order to re-connect with older, instinctive patterns of movement, which many of us have lost. We can make choices and rediscover the ease of movement we once had. Bodily memory has deeper evolutionary roots than factual memory. It enables us to acquire skills and know how to do things. Learning a physical skill takes time, and regular repetition is necessary. Once learned, the skill is not easily forgotten. There is increased brain activity in the

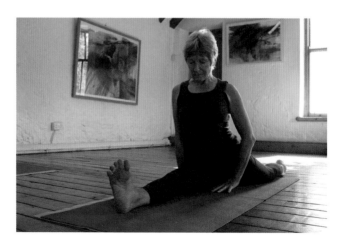

cerebral cortex during the learning phase, often experienced as concentrated effort and even frustration. The more variety we bring to the repetition of asana, the more enjoyable our learning can be. Once a skill becomes ingrained, it is gradually consolidated into the sub-cortical structures and becomes accessible.

Not only is it important to give clear, simple messages to your body with words and images, it is important to present them rhythmically in order to elicit a creative response. This repetition, aiming to be always clearer and more precise, intensifies the learning and the brain is rewired.

We approach our practice without taking anything for granted, realising that what we already 'know' is part of a much bigger picture.

F. M. Alexander,[11] whose technique has become widespread, refers to inhibition — the inhibition of ingrained, unhelpful habits. From the neuroscientific point of view, the capacity to choose not to do something is the essence of free will. When we stop and wait for the body's response, we are inhibiting the compulsions of reacting, doing, end-gaining or following another's authority; we give ourselves the freedom of choice. We choose to rediscover our natural movements by using our capacity for imagination.

When we are motivated to learn, the brain responds by creating order. We learn to stop using irrelevant muscles and to use those that are most efficient. We find more lightness, greater skill, more grace and relaxation. We gain a finer sensorial discrimination and our brain map becomes more precise.

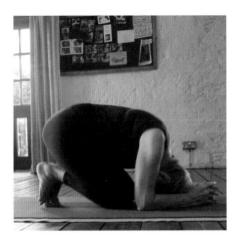 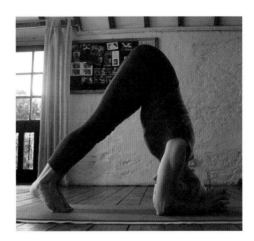

*'When a monkey does something, the neurons in its motor cortex fire in the characteristic pattern that shapes the behaviour in question. […] the motor neurons in a second monkey, who is **only passively** observing the behaviour of the first monkey, fire in the same pattern as those of the first monkey — thereby mirroring the observed behaviour "in imagination".'*

Solms and Turnbull[12]

This may explain why we can learn so much from watching another person whose skills we wish to absorb. At first, we don't know 'how' to look, or what exactly we are looking for. With the help of a teacher, our perception gradually changes and information seems to be passed from body to body.

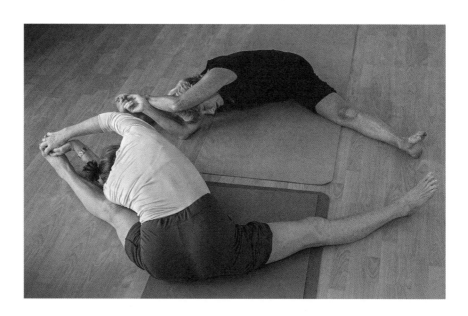

Elegant Architecture

'Posture attitudes of an animal are unconscious, while man's are largely determined by pre-conceived notions as to how he ought to look. The sensory-motor chain of reactions in our nerves and muscles has been gradually modified through association of ideas derived, not from mechanical or physical considerations of what balance means [...] but from moral, that is, social concepts.'

Mabel Todd[13]

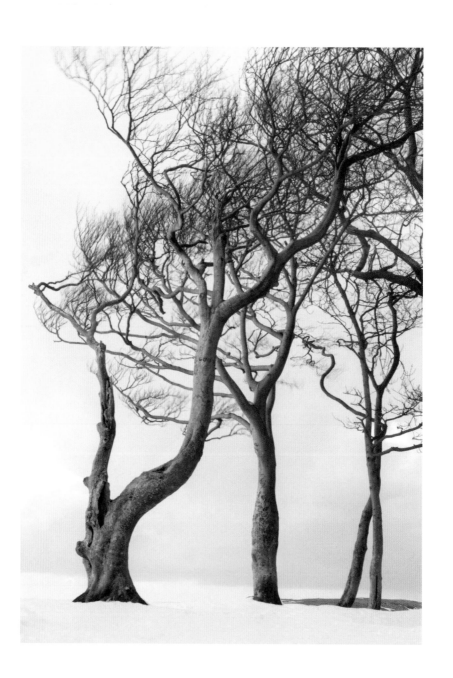

Intelligent Architecture

Considering the huge number of gestures, movements and positions the human body is capable of, most of us, especially in western culture, are extremely limited in our behaviour — so much so that, if we were to walk down the street with one hand placed on the back of the neck, or to squat on our seat on the bus, we would, no doubt, draw attention to ourselves. From the body's point of view, however, the 'norm' is very restrictive.

The architecture of the body reflects an intelligence that we will never grasp in its totality. Like all creatures, our bodies can be beautifully adapted to our environments — if we learn how to move with efficiency of effort. We can learn how to work with the body — not against it — and begin to realise how many of our usual habits disturb its innate harmony. It is not simply to have a practice of asana that we begin this yoga, but to bring the same intelligence to life when we walk, sit or stand, and when we bring our attention to the breath.

The human skeleton is not built for standing still. With its long fine limbs and many articulations, its primary function is movement. It looks as though it is made to dance.

The spine is the first part of the body to develop in the womb; the limbs start as buds and grow to, and then from, the spine. The rib-cage protects the lungs and the heart.

At birth the human spine has a C-shape. This shape changes as the infant begins to suckle, move, lift and turn, forming the first forward arch (cervical). From the instinctive movements of the legs pushing to, and away from the body, the second forward curve (lumbar) begins to appear, which will be formed during crawling, standing and walking.

Building Connections

Many of us, without realising it, are collapsed under our own weight. In this yoga practice, we become lighter by using our feet to move upward through our hips, connecting up through our spines; the internal architecture of the body asks to be acknowledged. We begin a new relationship with the breath.

The shoulder and hip joints are round: ball joints, capable of a wide range of movement. The way we use our arms and legs should not limit their movement or put stress on the spine. Ideally, the shoulder girdle floats and the pelvis is free, mediating the rebound from the ground and the pull of gravity. Hands and feet can delight in being the most articulated parts of the body.

As the large, superficial muscles relax and become less dominant, the deep, postural muscles are invited to play their part once again. These muscles are

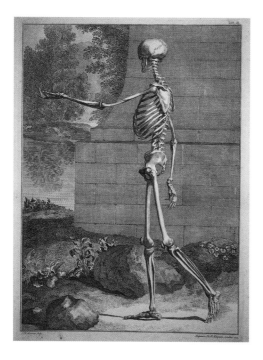
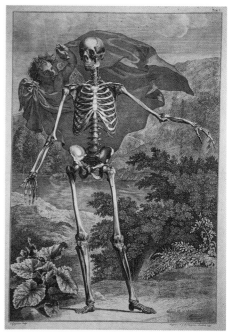

structured differently from the big locomotive ones and are harder to regain once they have fallen out of use. They are the muscles that a baby instinctively develops as it discovers how to support itself and to move; the muscles that an animal relies on for lightness and control.

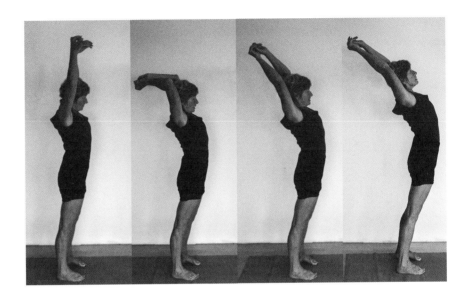

Machines can sometimes look very life-like, moving incrementally, making a series of small movements instead of one large movement. This is a key feature of an integrated yoga practice: moving not in one direction only, but in two opposite directions. This brings us closer to the source of the movement. Our actions take on a non-linear quality and become more pleasing.

Let us begin to see the aliveness of the spine. First of all, we have to let go of preconceptions, such as 'stretching', 'lengthening the spine', or 'being on the spine', which give us a fragmented sense of this vital core of the body. Any form of bracing prevents us from feeling the pathways within the body. As we release resistance, we discover a new spine. Each time a part of the spine comes alive, it is unexpected and new connections are revealed.

When we follow the architecture of the skeleton, we keep width between the tops of the thighs by working up from the outer edges of the feet, engaging the outer thigh muscles. This support from below allows us to relax the groins, buttocks, lower back and abdomen. The pelvis can then balance freely between the thighs and the spine.

> 'The arch is nothing else than a force originated by two weaknesses, for the arch in buildings is composed of two segments of a circle, each of which, being very weak in itself, tends to fall; but as each opposes this tendency in the other, the two weaknesses combine to form one strength.'
>
> Leonardo da Vinci[14]

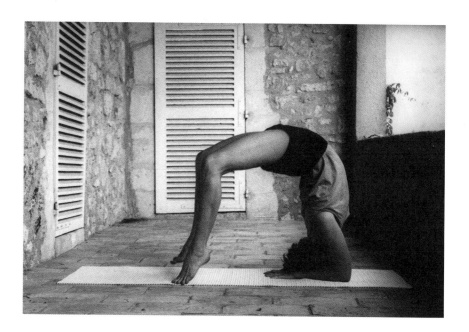

These arches are in our hands and feet, and in both the forward and backward curves of the spine. Through awareness of these arches, we can strengthen the working connections of each end of the arch.

As our practice develops, our movements acquire a new quality. We gain a new source of support and control; as if we are able to fly, yet can touch down to meet the ground at any moment. Then our contact with the ground is alive and strong — without heaviness. This is completely different from the usual interpretation of 'grounding'.

'In work of love, the body forgets its weight.
And once again with love and singing in my mind,
I come to what must come to me,
Carried as a dancer by a song.
This grace is gravity.'

Wendell Berry[15]

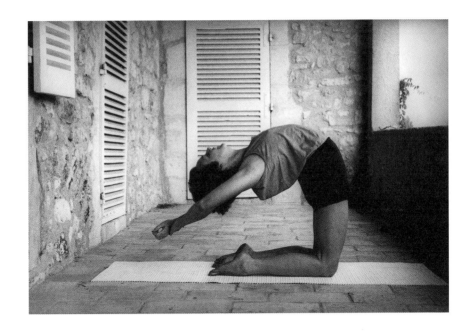

Questioning Asana

'When an asana comes about spontaneously as a natural expression of one's interior state, it will be perfect. That is to say, the position of legs, hands, arms, head, the gaze… everything will be as it should be…. Performance of an asana by an effort of will can never have the same perfection. Asanas are connected with the rhythm of one's breath, and the breath with one's state of mind at any particular time.'

Sri Anandamay[16]

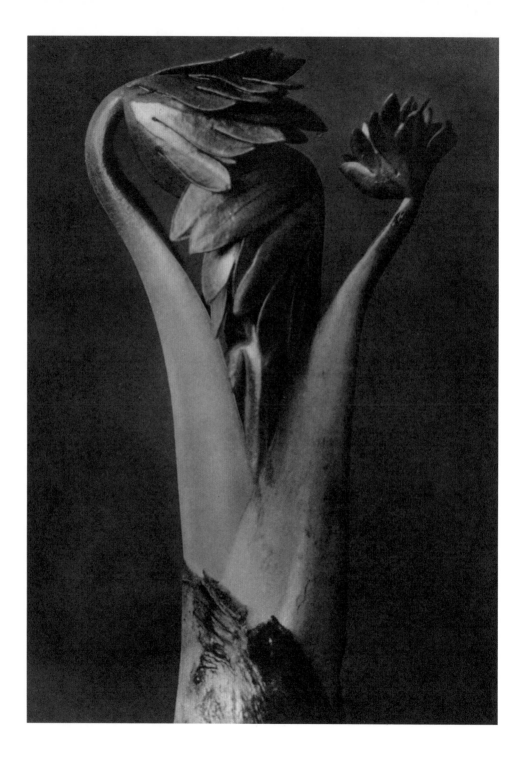

The Limitations of Language

Most students come to our classes with unhelpful habits or preconceived ideas about how asanas are done, just as we did when we started working with Vanda. Misunderstandings have even arisen from Vanda's own instructions and from statements in her book. She did not give explanations. Rather, she gave us direct experience through her hands and invited us to watch the movements in her body.

Examining, questioning and undoing habits becomes more interesting than step-by-step instructions. We become more innocent and gain new perspectives, finding different ways of approaching asanas.

When we first started to learn from Vanda, we had difficulty understanding her instructions. Yet we saw tremendous liveliness appear in the whole of her body in response to one specific adjustment.

Vanda used the least amount of effort. She emphasised the importance of certain details, but these details were to be understood in the context of the whole.

The process is difficult to describe and any attempts to do so are easy to misconstrue. It often happens that a descriptive phrase such as, 'the knees open' or 'the heels go down', is expressed or interpreted as an instruction: *'Open the knees!'* or *'Push the heels down!'* Misunderstanding is almost inevitable.

Remember, asanas do not have to look like themselves at first; only gradually do our bodies become more responsive and instructions easier to follow. Every part of the body needs to be addressed and felt. Some of Vanda's instructions are understood only after several years of practice.

For a few years, Vanda experimented with Tai Chi; she was interested in the similarities and the differences between the two practices.

> *'The energy is rooted in the feet*
> *Developed in the legs*
> *Directed by the waist*
> *And expressed through the fingers.*
> *— The feet, legs and waist must function as one unit.'*
> Zhang Sanfeng[17]

Her yoga was in agreement with this Tai Chi tenet except, for her, the knees were a vital part of this one functioning unit.

It is important to note that the suggestions in the following chapters represent only a few of the infinite number of connections that can come to life as we deepen our practice.

At times the text should have the feel of musical notation, inviting a sense of rhythm and playful investigation when practising.

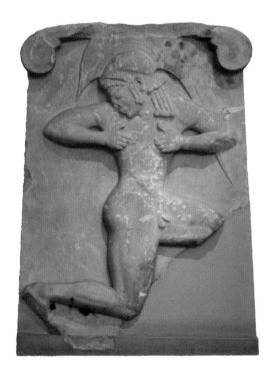

Clarifying Vanda's Instructions

There were certain phrases that Vanda often used. In this section, we have tried to unpack some of her 'sutras', so that you can experiment with them yourself.

'Yoga should be stress-free.'

Vanda was dedicated to developing a practice that did not stress the body; but this has often been misunderstood as gentle, effortless yoga. To discover how to be relaxed, and yet intensely alive, is hard work. What we think of as relaxation is often collapse which causes stress on joints, unrecognized until damage is done. To change our lazy ways takes effort; sometimes we can barely sustain the effort for more than a few seconds, as the muscles are learning to work in different ways.

'Lock the knees.' 'Stretch the knees.' 'Straighten the knees.'

We learn to engage the knee by finding out how to use the muscles of the foot and leg. Once the knee is engaged, space must be kept inside and around the joint. When Vanda straightened her knees, she did so after making a series of interconnected movements, without losing the connection from the heels that runs through the spine.

Try this:
In a standing position, engage the front and sides of the feet in front of the ankle; then use your heels to engage the knees. Be aware of the response in the upper body and lower spine.

Once you have accessed the awareness, try:
— moving from standing into wide legs;
— focusing on the knees in Dog Pose and Uttanasana; when you engage the knees appropriately, there can be so much space below the ankles that the heels do not want to lift;
— exploring the turning in and out capability of the ankles.

'Heels down.' 'Have weight in the heels.'

We do not push weight into the heels. Instead, by engaging the front part of the foot and ankle, the upper body becomes lighter. Then, we can travel through the centre of the foot towards the heels and the heels can engage to open the knees.

In preparation for a Backbend from the ground:
'Touch the back of the waist to the ground.'

Lying on the back with the knees bent, we engage the lower hips and outer thighs to invite a collecting towards the sacrum so, at first, the back of the waist comes away from the ground. Then, from the upper body, we connect with the heels. This invites the opening between the fourth and fifth lumbar vertebrae. Only then does the back rim of the pelvis spread and meet the floor. This has nothing to do with pushing the spine to the ground.

It takes time to find this action. It cannot be hurried, but it can be invited.

In sitting positions: *"Hips heavy and wide." "Let the weight sink down."*

When we use the word 'hips', we are referring to the area formed by the side of the pelvis and the upper part of the femur.

We never drop our weight helplessly downwards. Rather, we learn to differentiate and isolate muscles in the hip basin. The outer muscles relate to the legs, shoulders and arms. The inner pelvic muscles relate to the lower spine .

'Drop the chin into the little hole between
the collar bones at the base of the neck.'

There is an opposing and equally important connection made in the back, which helps the vertebrae fit more deeply into the base of the skull on either side of the spine. If both of these opposing movements are activated — one, and then the other — the cervical vertebrae are enlivened.

'Gravitate.' 'Roots down.' 'Let gravity take hold of your body.'

Letting gravity take hold of your body is not a passive action but a dynamic response. We must stay mindful of the separation in the middle of the spine. Vanda often said, *'always go up to go down and always go down to go up.'*

'The muscles of the thighs are like iron.'

The outer thighs are the conduit between the hips and the ground so they do become more toned and firm. When the heels pull the knees open, you then discover the inner thigh muscles, which lead from the knees upward through the lower spine. This helps the femur joint stay more articulate. It means working with one group of muscles at a time.

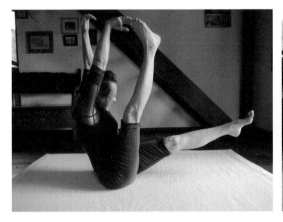
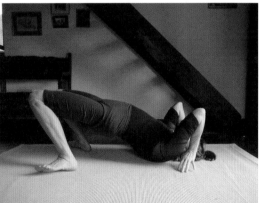

'The Egyptian spine was completely straight.'

The word 'straight' is misleading here. Vanda was speaking of the spine lengthening through its own connections, resulting in a sensation of the spine being straightened.

There can be a correspondence between the lumbar and cervical curves. The muscles on each side of these forward curves — not the curves themselves — lengthen when the top and bottom of the spine are deeply engaged. This is not a held position, nor a straightening of the spine. It is a rhythmical pattern of activity and release.

In forward bends: *'Drop the back of the lower spine to the floor.'*

There is more subtlety to this than first appears. A separation occurs in the back of the waist and an opposing separation in the front of the waist. The separation in the back of the waist gives lightness to the upper body and thighs.

Then we can engage the thighs, noticing the separation between coccyx and sacrum. The coccyx has unravelled without pulling the sacrum down.

'Tighten', 'Squeeze' or 'Press the thighs.'

This does not describe a holding of the thigh muscles. It refers to a rhythmical letting go and engagement of the outer thigh muscles.

'Follow the wave of the breath.'

Each breath asks for an alert renewal of attention. The wave of the exhalation is upwards, away from the ground; the wave of the inhalation is expansive. The spine becomes more alive and energy moves upwards.

'Three friends: breath, gravity and the wave.'

These friends are more elusive than they sound. By latching on to superficial interpretations we are likely to interfere with profound harmonious connections within the body. Discovering the meaning of these concepts takes time and patience. The wave is not a vague surge of energy upon which we ride in an asana — rather it is a series of incremental wave-like impulses resulting in movement. Befriending the breath requires waking up the body to the possibilities of more freedom and lightness. Gravity is harnessed more intelligently as we cultivate the division between the fourth and fifth lumbar vertebrae.

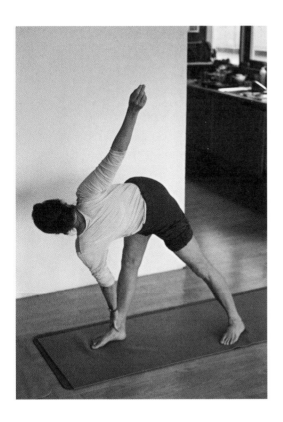
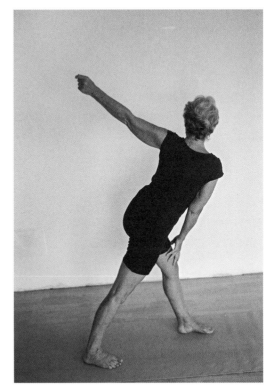

When walking: *'Allow the heel to make initial contact with the ground.'*

The heel is more than the back part of the foot. If you experiment with walking backwards one step at a time, paying attention, you become aware of what taking a step forward can be.

Try this:

— with one foot forward —

— the knee can help engage the front of the front foot on the ground —

— then, without the knee, engage the front of the front foot, on the ground —

— now walk from the heel of the front foot

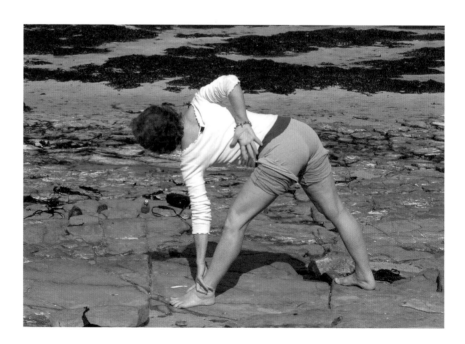

Assumptions About Practice

Diane

Once, Vanda was trying to help me open my very tight knees by developing their connection with the heels. After a summer away from my teacher, I returned to my first lesson in the autumn, eager to show her my progress, quite pleased with my understanding. I entered the small room with the piano and large mirror to find Vanda standing on two twigs and pointing to another two. *'That is your branch of the tree. You alight and take flight from it. We are not women, we are birds.'* So began a whole new exploration of the body's inner connections. My old way of learning, with diligence and concentration, was tossed out of the window, yet again. I had to take detours and bring in the element of surprise for my body to wake up. This meant rearranging myself to become a bird, discovering how, and with what speed, to move and how to find rest.

Many styles and schools of yoga have fixed principles, to which practitioners are asked to adhere in their practice and training. Many of these principles are ultimately limiting and, therefore, unhelpful to the continued expansion of a lifelong yoga practice. Here we address some of these principles and assumptions, and explain why they are unnecessary.

The body must be aligned

Animals and the rest of nature are not concerned about alignment. Why restrict the body? We follow the map of the body with as much precision as possible, in order to find ease of movement. Alignment would be an artificial imposition.

Yoga positions are often asymmetrical situations, which require a subtle and refined apprehension of wholeness.

There are exercises for 'opening' our hips

A common misunderstanding is that we can gain greater flexibility in the hips by spreading the legs wide and stretching the inner thighs to pull the inner groins open; or sitting in Baddha Konasana with the knees falling outwards, and trying to push the knees down and out.

This type of exercise comes from a fragmented intent, without reference to the spine or the joints. Do not make these forced movements.

The lower spine is contained within the hips. Both the outer hips and the outer thighs must engage in order to lighten and connect the lower spine upwards. This enlivens the feet, and the relationship between feet and hips becomes clearer.

Stretching is essential

We have many layers of muscles. Conscious stretching risks engaging only the large muscles, and causing tension elsewhere. Why put our attention on stretching the surface muscles only? This prevents us from becoming aware of deeper muscle connections.

The breath can be used in order to relax, or controlled to coincide with movements

The breath is not a tool. It responds and changes as our understanding and use of the body changes. Make sure that you do not force or hold the breath.

Counter-poses are necessary to counteract the effects of previous asanas

When we worked with Vanda it became obvious that there was no reason to follow Backbends with forward bends. Every position was approached according to the same principles, and the concept of counter-pose was irrelevant. When we practise well, we neither stretch nor overstretch and there is nothing to redress.

Balance is a priority

Trying to maintain balance causes tension. While we rearrange the body around the spine, we may need to lose our balance until a new balance is discovered. This is an on-going process and may take a long time.

There are no fixed points in the body that take weight. The part of the body in contact with the ground is alive and lightness comes from that contact. Remember that all parts of the body work in concert.

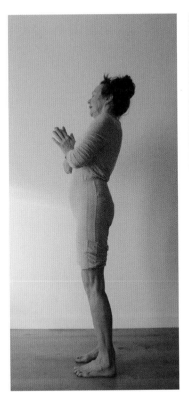
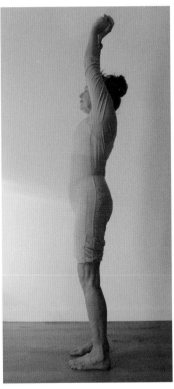
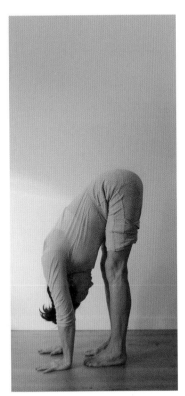

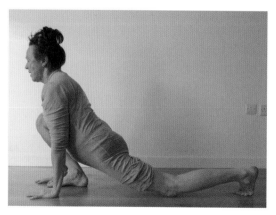 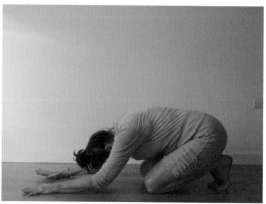

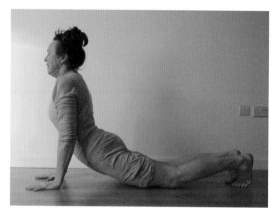 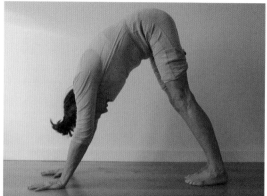

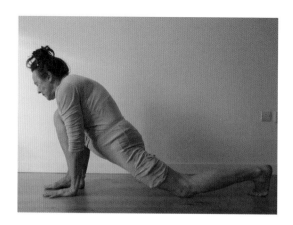

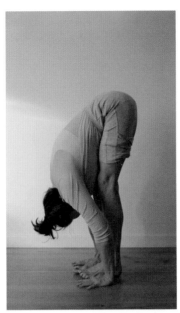

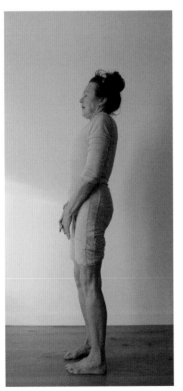
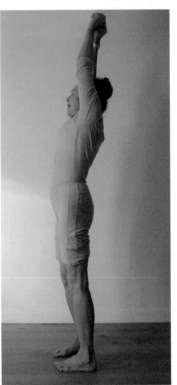
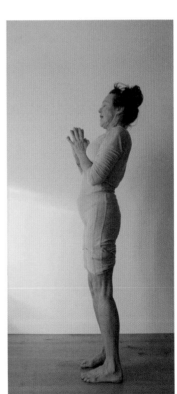

Habits

When Albert Hash, a fiddle maker in the Appalachian mountains, was asked how he made such beautiful instruments, he replied, *'Ain't nothing to it. You just take away all the wood that ain't fiddle, and you got yourself a fiddle.'*

We refine and simplify our practice, learning to let go of superfluous habits, mental and physical, which prevent us from exploring and being creative. It can take years to be able to make a simple movement, such as raising an arm, with integrity and elegance. Vanda's only explanation for the adjustments she made to our practice was, *'because it is more beautiful'*. It took time for us to appreciate the truth of this, though we could see it in the ease and harmony of her movements.

The following are the most common unhelpful habits we see in our students, and some suggestions for redressing them.

Undirected movement

We sometimes see students wiggling around or shaking their limbs, often an interpretation of the instruction to undo tension.

Why is this unhelpful? Because our attention is taken away from the spine. Our focus should be on greater precision.

Break the habit: Any gesture that we make in preparation for asana or during asana should be well considered and well executed.

When sitting, using the 'sitting' bones as a point of reference

Some students even pull out the gluteus muscles so as to sit more securely on the bones.

Why is this unhelpful? The ischial tuberosities should not be part of the focus of our attention. To use them as a base for sitting interferes with opening into, and through, the middle of the spine, losing the lightness and freedom of the upper body — arms, shoulders, neck, head.

Break the habit: Learn from a pre-school child about how to stand from sitting.

Sit, with crossed legs, as if about to stand up — without leverage or pulling — using your hands to lift your weight off your hips — even to lift yourself off the ground.

Now, engage your feet and thighs — sitting, with crossed legs, dropping deeply through the hips — let the back of the skull bring the lower spine — bit by bit — through the thighs, away from the heels.

Spreading fingers and toes on the ground

Why is this unhelpful? This causes us to lose the integrity of the hands and feet. It is important to keep palms and soles alive through their arches so that the wrists and ankles are spacious and free to rotate.

Break the habit: When standing, use the balls of the feet to invite the weight of the toes back through the ankles; in this way the heel is rested. Observe how the ankle rotates. Then, from the back of the heel, bring the weight of the toes forward through the ankle, engaging the heel. Observe how the ankle changes its rotation.

In Uttanasana, try making light fists of the hands as they touch the floor, bending the knees if touching the floor is not possible, so that the wrists become important for resting down through the arms. Now, the shoulders can both bring the spine forward, away from the heels, and rest the spine through the heels. When you open the hands, they will work differently.

Fixing the pelvis

Why is this unhelpful? If the pelvis is fixed, it prevents us from giving our attention to the spine within the hips. The connection between the light upper body and the developing strength of the lower body is inhibited. You will limit and create strain in the shoulder and hip joints.

Break the habit: Remember that the pelvis has a slight tilt forward around the middle of the spine and a slight tilt backward just above the femur bones.

Starting with the back foot — find the pathway towards the back of the skull — through the spine.

Starting with the front foot — find the connection towards the back of the skull — through the spine.

The hips are now a container for the lower spine — from the feet find the pathway — upwards through the shoulders into the arms.

Misuse of the base of the asana: the connection with the ground

In Headstand

Preparing the base by spreading the hands on the floor, or clutching the head with the hands, or forcing the elbows to match the width of the shoulders.

Why is this unhelpful? In all these cases, the shoulders are unable to have freedom of movement, which causes strain on the cervical vertebrae. As a result it is impossible to move into headstand without pulling or pushing, which compromises the cervical vertebrae even more, and creates rigidity in pelvis and legs.

Break the habit: The base of headstand should not be inert or rigid — there can be a division and distribution of weight.

First, resting the hips' weight down through head and wrists — then, directing from the hands — shoulders can carry the spine's weight upwards, away from the head, while the head is dropping its weight into the ground — hands, alternately, relax and engage.

And now, hands planting elbows into the ground — hands planting forearms into the ground — yet, shoulders carrying weight into the hips — shoulders carrying weight to the feet.

Pushing the feet into the ground in Dog Pose, Backbends and Standing poses

Why is this unhelpful? It compromises the shoulder, hip and elbow joints, reducing lightness and articulation in the upper body, making the body tighter and stiffer.

Break the habit: Shift the centre of gravity upward, above the centre of the spine. Freeing the shoulders, drop your feet. Now, beginning from the hands, engage the feet.

Pushing with the feet in Urdhva Dhanurasana

Why is this unhelpful? If we push and pull with the legs, we create tension in the lower back, neck and shoulders.

Break the habit: In preparation for Urdhva Dhanurasana, connect your hips towards your shoulders until your elbows are free, then connect your hips towards your head until your hands come alive. Now, from your feet, engage through your legs into the hips.

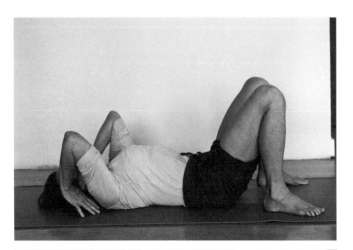

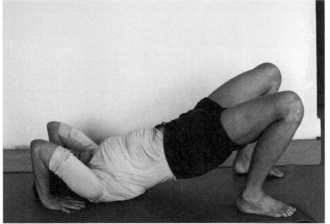

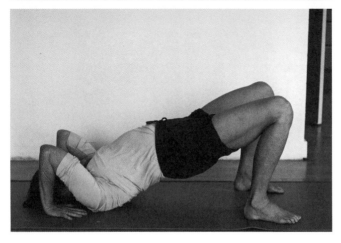

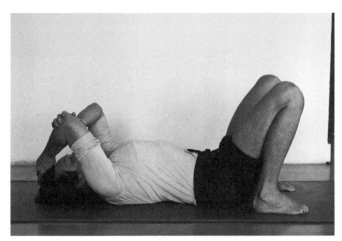

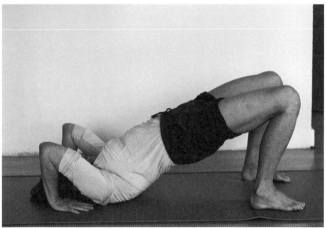

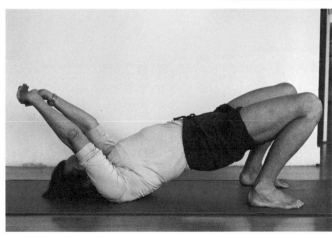

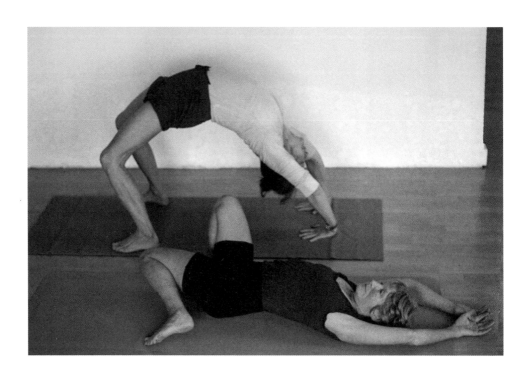

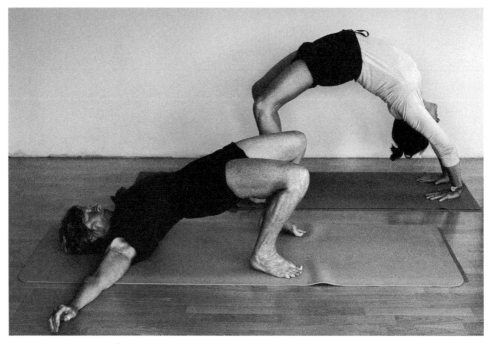

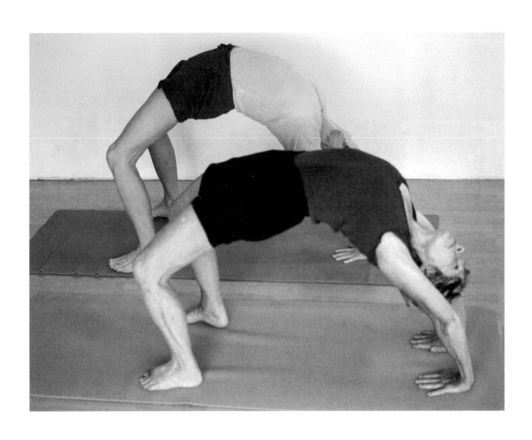

Pulling with the feet in inverted poses

Why is this unhelpful?

We lose the effectiveness of the base of the position, which is our control for moving in and out of, as well as remaining in, the asana. Without this responsive base, tension is pulled into the shoulders and too much weight is taken by the cervical spine.

Break the habit: Instead, use your knees or thighs to send your feet away.

Pushing away from the hands in Dog Pose and in preparation for Headstand or Shoulderstand

Why is this unhelpful? It interferes with the deepening connection from the middle of the spine towards the base of the skull and the opposing, and equally important, connection from the heels to the middle of the spine.

Break the habit: Refuse to push — and see what happens.

In Shoulderstand, pulling the shoulders together for a higher lift

Why is this unhelpful? It forces the legs up and doesn't allow for any deep connection within the back of the spine, or any deep connection into the base of the skull — which creates an unequal relationship between the front and back of the spine.

Break the habit: Create a widening base between the shoulders, yet also try to keep the top of the shoulders on the ground. In this way the arms can be free to play their part more effectively. Do not be afraid to let the thoracic spine bow outwards at first. Then, from above, the outer feet and thighs send the base of the spine downwards to make a deeper connection with, and into, the middle of the spine. It is now possible to correct the outward bow of the thoracic spine and the whole spine feels light and lifted.

In Shoulderstand, using the hands to support the back or obtain more lift
Why is this unhelpful? It places a great deal of strain on the neck.

Break the habit: The goal is not to send the spine up through the sacrum, but to let the sacral area rest into the fourth and fifth lumbar spine.

Remember not to hurry into the position. Take your time. Before putting your arms behind your back, try moving them into different positions — up in the air, out to the sides, behind your head. This helps to rediscover the base, so that the hands are not disconnected from the rest of the body. Leverage is not the primary objective.

Head, elbows and shoulders are the base of this asana. Vanda called it neck-balance, the neck forming the bridge between the top of the shoulders and head.

Spacing feet and legs far apart in standing positions
Why is this unhelpful? It tends to make one stretch and brace the legs, creating tension in the upper body.

Break the habit: Begin with your feet about hip width apart and slowly increase the distance between them. Notice how your feet can stay light and articulate. There is less bracing and locking of the legs, less distortion around knees and ankles. This brings more freedom and lightness to the upper body.

In Virabhadrasana, keeping the bent knee aligned with the ends of the toes
Why is this unhelpful? Trying to keep the knee fixed causes tension and fragmentation.

Break the habit: Draw weight up, away from the legs. Engage from the back foot up through the back leg so that both spine and front knee feel their freedom upwards. You can rely on the very back of the back heel as the front knee releases forward. Then the front heel descends to engage the front knee.

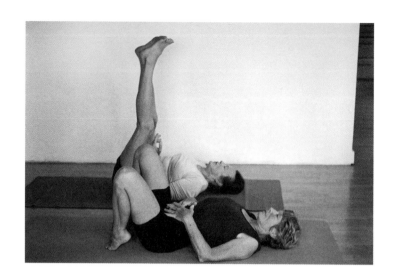

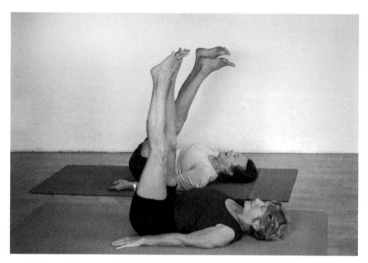

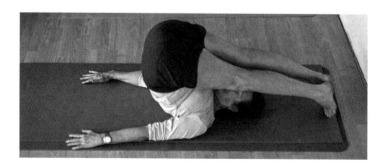

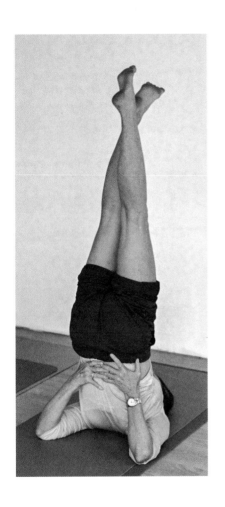

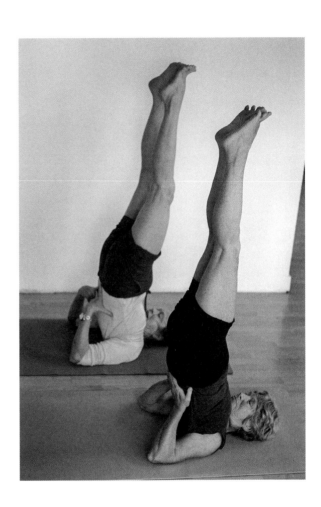

Locking or over-stretching the knees; keeping the knees bent

Why is this unhelpful? Both these habits restrict mobility in the knee, ankle and hip joints. Injuries to knees, hips and tendons of the lower leg are extremely common and it is important to understand how to use the feet, ankles and knees in a healthy way.

Break the habit: Avoid straightening your legs until you have a clearer understanding of how the leg works in relation to the rest of the body. On the other hand, don't keep your knees permanently bent. Use the foot in such a way as to keep the knee slightly rotational, both inwards and outwards. Try not to lose this when you engage the heel.

Using props

Why is this unhelpful? In sitting positions, using blocks and blankets to tilt the pelvis forward, or using a belt to pull oneself forward, compromises the freedom of the femur joints and wrists, and shortens the front of the spine. Placing blankets under the neck and shoulders to do shoulderstand does not protect the neck. The head and neck are an integral and active part of the posture and should not be separated from the rest of the body. Head, elbows and shoulders need to be on the same plane. The spine unrolls from the coccyx through the sacrum into the lumbar area and, with the elbows kept down, the cervical vertebrae become an alive bridge between head and shoulders.

Break the habit: Props are a lazy way out of a problem unless used very creatively.

— Question their use if it inhibits you from finding deep connections within the body.
— Question the use of props if the intent is merely to achieve the asana.
— Question the use of props if it involves pushing or pulling.
— Question why you are doing the asanas.

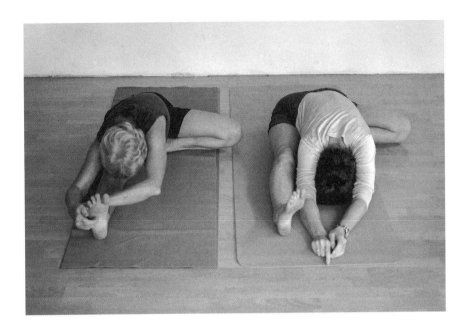

Through enquiry and practice, we begin to glimpse another way of being in our body, which we recognise as being true to the way it is made. However effortful it seems, the body is grateful and feels refreshed as though it has come home to itself.

If our practice can be imbued with rhythm and a quiet, receptive attitude, a dialogue is established in which waiting for the body's response is just as important as performing the action.

Rethinking Anatomy

'While doing the poses correctly our muscles seem to answer to a binding force collecting them together. This force, responding to the opposite pull of gravity, travels through our limbs and is well accepted by our body, which naturally desires to extend itself.'

Vanda Scaravelli[18]

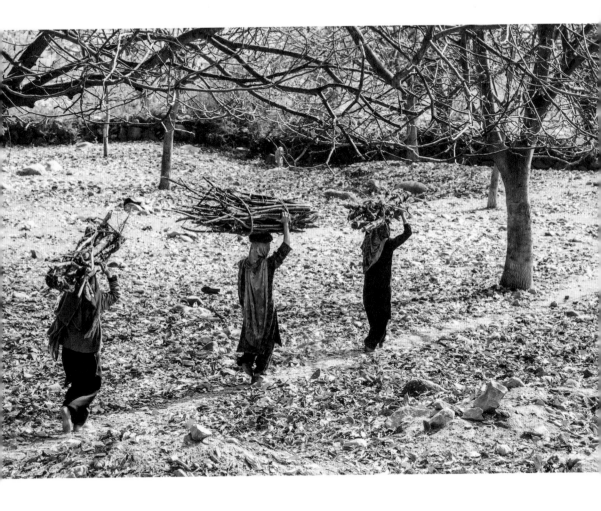

Finding Freedom

There is wisdom to be received from the body, a memory of lightness and simple symmetry from the time when we were forming and moving within a fluid environment. One can regain and recall this sense.

As we swim upwards through the spine to discover the rhythm of the lungs, we find more freedom, more connections. We learn to trust the intelligence of the body as we explore these connections, particularly those which lead us back to the spine. We learn our anatomy from experience, based on the reality of muscles, bones, nerves and joints. This science of open-ended exploration leads us towards the magic of the body.

Would a tiger move more efficiently if it understood its own anatomy? Would an infant learn better how to walk if the process could be explained to her? A conventional teaching of anatomy may interfere with the development of an intuitive and experiential relationship with the body.

The body keeps redefining itself; when one part becomes more intelligent, other parts change and rearrange themselves. Every place is as good as any other to start our mapping and pathway finding. Questions will arise which challenge the obvious. This may create resistance or discordance. However, later on, greater freedom and understanding will result.

Ask some questions of your body:
— Which is the longest bone?
— Which is the largest joint? The heaviest joint?
— Where are your ball-and-socket joints?
— What are the segments of the spine?

Then pose questions to these parts of your body, one at a time:
— How do you connect from above and from below?
— How do you carry or transfer weight through?

Experiment, like a child playing with Lego or piecing a jigsaw together. You can begin to assemble clues and insights from this attention and it may be easier to mobilise your imagination. Explore with curiosity so that you do not settle for easy or automatic answers; find words that match your discoveries.

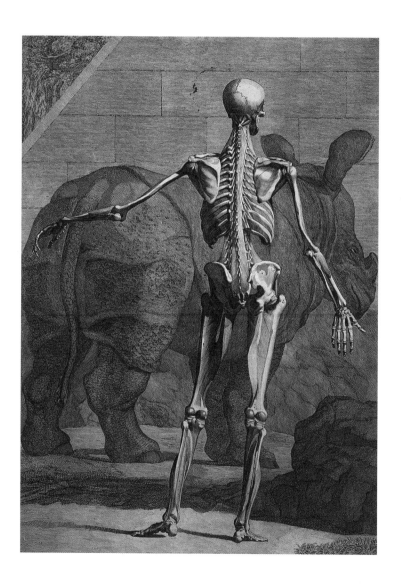

Rethinking the Spine and Pelvis

There are always new ways of seeing and defining the spine. The spine can rearrange itself as it comes alive, bit by bit. Every new encounter is a surprise and cannot be predicted from our factual knowledge. Pushing, pulling and forcing can be replaced with muscles relaying movement throughout the spine. The spine can rest itself and then lighten itself, giving the lungs greater freedom.

In *Awakening the Spine,* Vanda speaks of a revolution:

> 'A division in the centre of our back, where the spine moves simultaneously in two opposite directions: from the waist down, towards the legs and feet, which are pulled by gravity, and from the waist upwards, through the top of the head, lifting us up freely.'[19]

Before we can discover this, it is necessary to make friends with the spine in new ways. Here are some suggestions.

The ends of the spine

Begin to free both ends of the spine. Relax the top cervical vertebra, releasing the head away from the feet. We can begin to understand how tension around the skull, the lower jaw area and the top of the sternum interferes with mobility.

The sacrum carries a memory of movement in its four or five, lightly fused, small vertebrae. The coccyx can eventually unfurl away from the sacrum if the muscles of the inner groins, pubic and hip joints release tension. When we permit more space in the pubic joint, the slight opening allows bones to realign. We can retain mobility into old age.

The relationship between the skull and the pelvis

The skull is able to tilt forward and backward around the top of the spine. The pelvis tilts slightly forward around the centre of the spine and backward around the femur joints. This harmonious relationship allows the weight of the head to rest the spine without falling onto it and allows one to work deeply into the large lumbar and smaller cervical vertebrae at the same time.

Respecting the lumbar and cervical curves

The lumbar and cervical curves do not straighten. The muscles on either side of them lengthen and the deeper muscles expand.

There can be a lengthening up through the sacral spine, while the shoulders keep the upper spine rested. Then, as the head keeps the spine rested, there is a widening from the centre of the spine. This creates more space and movement in the sacral and thoracic (dorsal) spine.

— The cervical curve rests towards the lumbar curve —
 which lightens upwards in response.
— The lumbar curve rests upwards towards the cervical curve —
 which lightens in response.
— A lively dance goes on between them —
 up and down throughout the spine.

A memory is awakened in the pelvis, whose muscles can come to life in a different way. Often, we allow the muscles of the legs and buttocks to dominate, but it is the pelvic muscles that wish to regain this honour. The pelvis is never fixed; it stays free to accommodate the rebound from the ground up through the legs. After all, we don't try to fix the position of the pelvis when running or dancing.

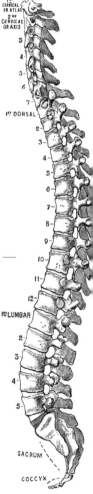

82

The segments of the spine

The spine relates to itself through its segments, like a snake. If a cobra were grasped by the back of its hood, thus deprived of the ability to attack, it would try to escape by making incremental movements from its tail upwards.

As another example, when we twirl around, there is a sense of the spine releasing upwards through its segments. When we pause, the spine connects back downward. The feet can regain the memory of the upward release.

Connecting through the centre of the spine

Connecting the spine through the centre is a natural action, which most of us have lost. Harnessing gravity does not begin with pushing the feet down. It begins with having, as a focal point, the division in the back of the spine, the area around the fifth lumbar vertebra, where the weight from the spine above falls. This weight needs to be redirected upwards. Then the pelvic muscles just inside the hips can become engaged.

In a separate endeavour, we can redirect the weight upwards through the front of the fifth lumbar area. A deeper, stronger impetus is needed to engage the muscles upward along the front of the spine inside the pelvis.

There are endless perspectives for exploring the spine:
— What does your spine look like?
— What does your spine feel like?
— Where does it begin?
— Where does it end?
— Can you sense your spine without your arms and legs?
— Which parts of your spine are heavy? Which are light?
— Ask the same questions sitting, lying and standing.

How the thighs relate to the pelvis and spine

Once we have established lightness in the upper body, we can start to engage from below. Outer thighs and feet become important in directing movement through the pelvis. As the front of the foot remains deeply engaged into the ground, the lightness of the upper body is not disturbed.

Try resting your hands on a surface to invite a lightening upwards through the spine. This happens through the hips and through the shoulders.

Engage your feet with the ground to invite a movement upward through the sacrum, first the back of the sacrum, and then the front. Come back to the resting hands to give life to the spine. Continue to repeat rhythmically.

When the outer thigh muscles take weight away from the hips, the inner thigh muscles take weight away from the inner knee and create space in the pubic joint. From the heels below, we are able to open up around the knee joint.

Now, try the previous practice again, keeping these two actions in mind.

The gluteus muscles learn to stop pushing and gripping. This gives more freedom to the muscles around the sacral area. In time, the pelvic floor muscles become more effective for participation in breathing.

It is essential not to try too hard, for then the effort would be directed by muscles which are already over-used. Keep a clear image of what you're doing. The work must be simple if the results are to be strong, deep and clear.

Spine and breathing

We harness gravity and work with it through the centre of our spine. Enlivening the spine improves breathing, which benefits every organ in the body, including the brain.

Balancing and re-balancing your weight, move your centre of gravity upwards. Rest and, then again, balance and re-balance your weight. Move it upwards once again. There is a complementary rhythm in breathing — two different actions and two different groups of muscles: one for inhalation and another for exhalation.

In time, the action of breathing has the quality of a bird flying — the shoulders release their arms and the spine releases its lungs as arms.

The head and neck

The neck is an erect, curved and moving column for the load of the head.

The head sits on the spine at a point just behind the articulation of the jaw, in line with the entrance to the ears. It rocks on a little cradle at the centre of its base. It is important for the proprioceptive system that the head is centred and not held up by muscular force.

The head weighs between ten and twenty pounds (4.5-5 kg). The muscles of the head, neck and jaw are very strong. Holding one's head off-centre causes strains throughout the spine.

As the spine becomes more alive in all its parts, the head and neck start to feel lighter and freer. The muscles feel balanced and less at risk of strain. We can begin to play with the weight of the head in various positions.

The instruction to pull the shoulders away from the ears that is often given in yoga classes can cause tension in the neck and limit freedom in the jaw and head. When the shoulder-girdle is brought back to its light connection with the head, both head and neck can become free.

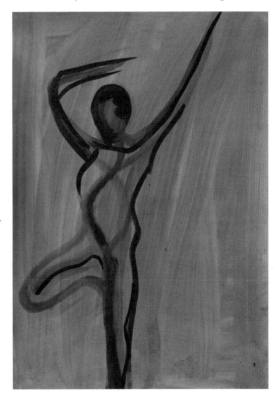

Students with neck tension or past injuries are often afraid to practise Shoulderstand and Headstand. They may have been warned against doing so by previous teachers and this adds to their anxiety.

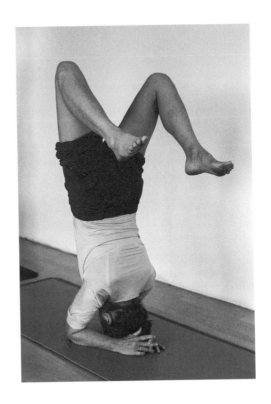

Diane

For a period of time, I developed deep pain and discomfort in my neck. I was told not to practise Headstand or Shoulderstand, but that did not seem to be a satisfactory answer. It seemed to me that the yoga asanas should be able to help me relieve this pain, but only if I worked very carefully, from the beginning, in order to understand each step towards an asana. This led me to understand better the relationships throughout the upper body and, separately, the lower body. Then I discovered how the two interacted with each other to produce an antigravity lightness through the spine. I discovered more movement around the coccyx than around the sacrum. To my surprise, the tension and pain in my neck abated. If I had stopped practising these two asanas, I would not have been taken on this fruitful journey.

Bandhas

The bandhas are parts of the body where tension is often held: the base of the spine and groins, the middle of the spine, and the top of the spine. The names of the bandhas corresponding with these areas are Moola bandha, Uddiyana bandha and Jalandara bandha, respectively. Mahabandha, or great bandha, is a balanced combination of all three.

There are many definitions of the word bandha. Often it is translated as 'lock' or 'knot'; however, it is also translated as 'redirect', 'catch' or 'build a bridge over the sea'.

Though Vanda did not refer to the bandhas in her teaching, we were brought to sense their importance. Her focus of attention was the spine, which she recognised as the source of all movements.

When the spine becomes the central focus of our practice and the middle of the spine develops its importance, the bandhas release their tension and the body finds new or forgotten connections. Gradually, with practice, these new connecting movements deepen and strengthen.

When the Mahabandha is achieved, a subtle process goes on within the deeper layers of the body, mapped in traditional yoga literature as the system of chakras. Vanda used different language. She talked of awakening the spine and bringing more life through the fourth and fifth lumbar area — the revolution she refers to in her own book.

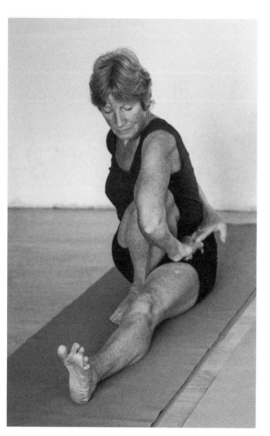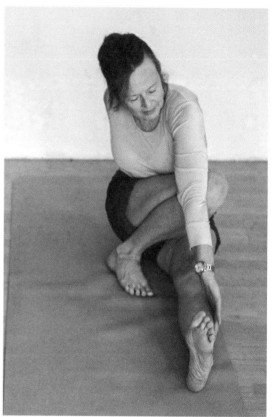

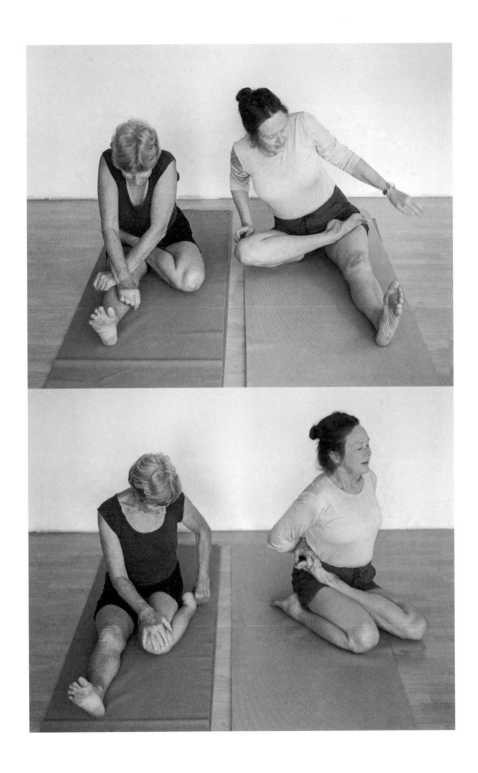

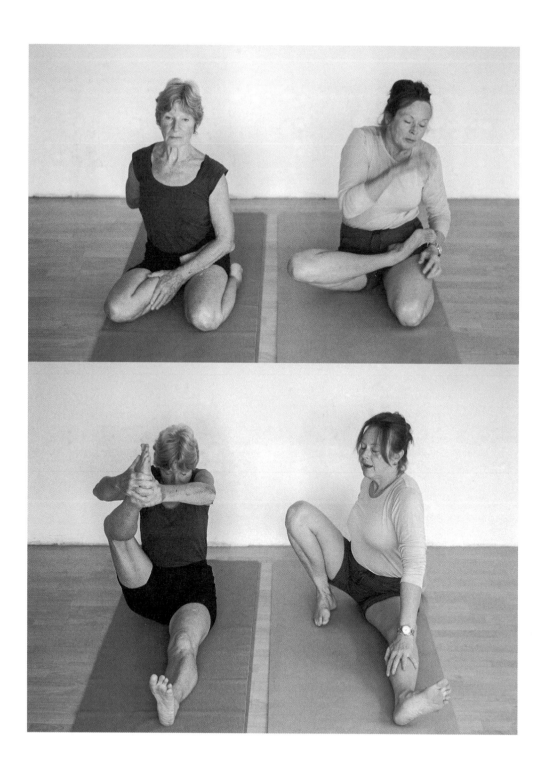

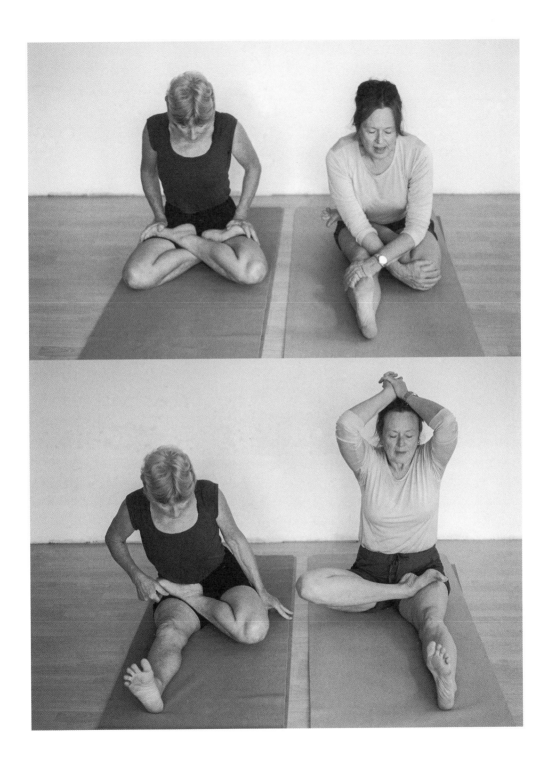

The Joints

We enjoy movement thanks to our joints, but they often become sites of tension. When practising yoga, it is important to think of their range of motion and quality of articulation. When they work efficiently, movements are more graceful.

The relationship between the thigh and shoulder joints is fundamental to the awakening of the spine.

When we sit, stand or walk, weight from the upper body falls onto the lower spine and femur joints. Because the latter are deeper and tighter than the shoulder joints, they are less mobile. Be sure to give them as much space and freedom as possible.

Find the connection between the femur and shoulder joints through the front centre of the spine; you can then discover a similar connection through the back centre of the spine.

Try sitting with your legs apart. If you find that the weight of your legs prevents you from feeling these connections, cross your ankles to discover them.

Now try nestling your arms close to your body like folded wings. Again the connection between shoulder and femur joints is felt.

The knees

The knee is a hinging and rotating joint. It is the largest in the body and orchestrates the connections between the foot and the femur joint (sometimes called the hip joint) and between the heel and upper body. It is often experienced as vulnerable because it is asked to take more than its share of the weight. It is up to us to educate the leg, so that we can use it more efficiently.

When standing, by working from the ground upwards, we can use the feet to discover the upper end of the lower leg bones just below the knee. The outer bone of the lower leg (tibia) is the nearest to vertical of all the bones in the body. We can strengthen the connection from ankle to knee to straighten and lengthen the tibia. Only then, through the rotation of muscles around the inner bone of the lower leg (fibula), can the heels open the knees. This helps keep the knee spacious and rotational from below.

Imagine looking forward from behind the kneecap. It is all too easy to push the knee back or keep it held between tight muscles in the upper and lower legs.

Once we have refined and understood these articulations in the lower part of the body, there will be less reactive tension from below when we bring our attention to the upper body.

The shoulders

The ball and socket joint of the shoulder has a wide range of movement and many connections to be discovered.

We use our hands all the time, usually without any awareness of their connection with the shoulders. Keep your shoulders free and let them find their own response to the movements of your hands.

Try each of the following, staying aware of your shoulders:
— Keeping your hands relaxed, as if they don't know what will be asked of them, bring the palms together in a gesture of prayer. Shoulders free.
— Now rest your hands, palms down, to touch a surface. Shoulders free.
— Now take your arms up in the air and release upwards beyond your hands. Shoulders free.
— Now bring your hands together to clap. Shoulders free.
— Now mime eating with your hands. Shoulders free!

We can discover much movement in the upper body, both towards and away from the spine. Remember that the shoulder blades hang from the sides of the chest as well as from the back. This potential freedom of the muscles of the shoulder blades and the area around the clavicle is necessary for giving the shoulder its full range of movement. The shoulder joint is connected to every bone in the trunk of the body.

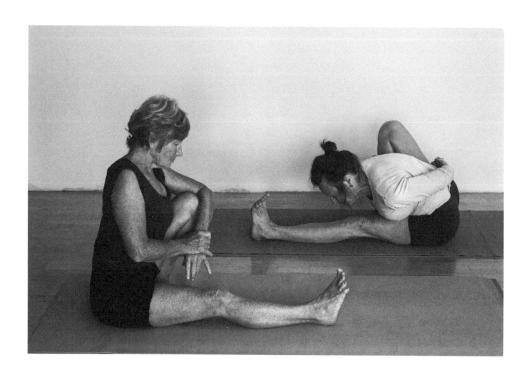

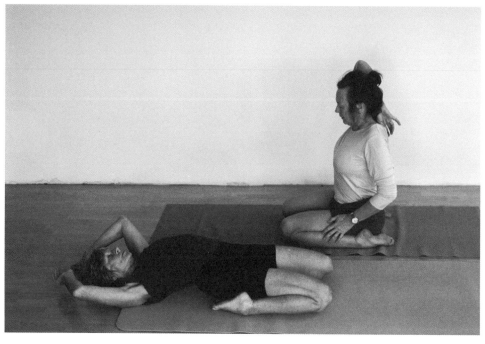

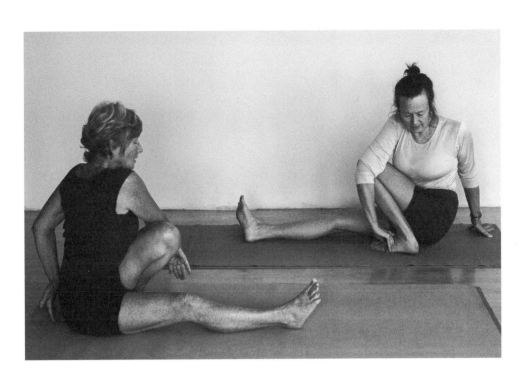

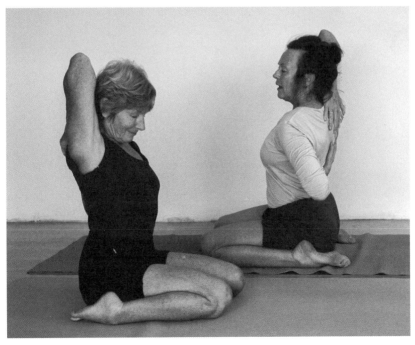

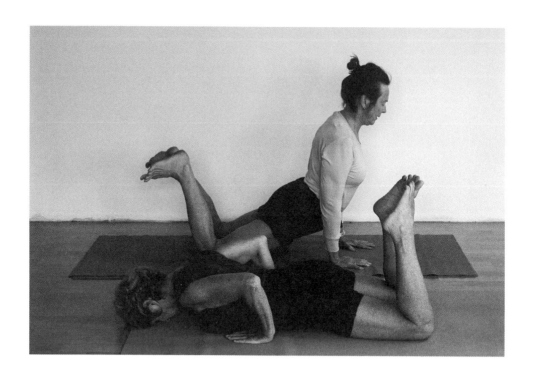

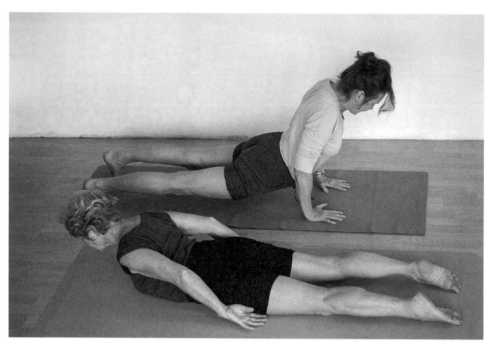

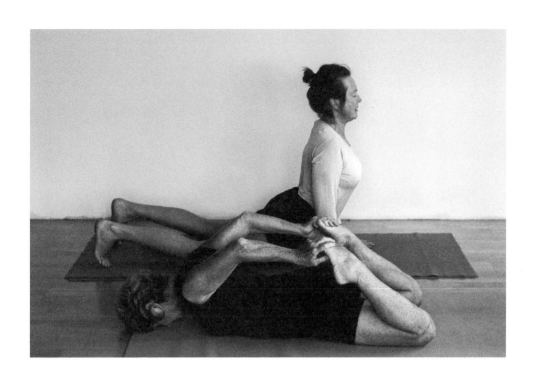

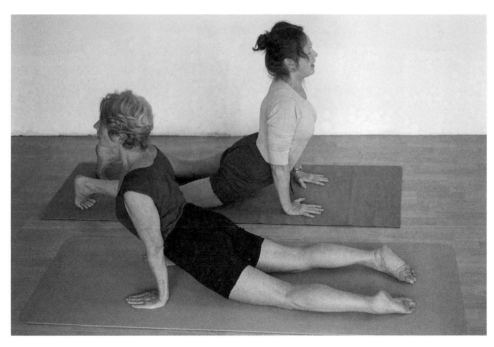

The torso has a complex arrangement of muscles:
— around the ribs
— from spine to sternum
— through the entire length of the back
— attached to every vertebra from the skull to the sacrum
— to the strong muscle bands of the front abdominal wall
— to the pelvis

We learn to respect this multi-layered, multi-directional arrangement of muscles in order to find greater efficiency in our movements and in breathing.

Try each of the following, staying aware of your shoulders:
— Ask the shoulder and chest area to stay quiet — even when the arms are making strong gestures.
— In Headstand, give weight from the lower spine and through the back to the shoulders, without collapsing them. The shoulders, which are now weight-bearing, can send you through the arms. Give the weight of your head to the ground. Hands and shoulders can now take the cervical spine up, away from your head, which continues to rest into the ground.
— In Shoulderstand, from the base of the spine, the shoulders define themselves on the ground. Through the lumbar spine, the shoulders again define themselves on the ground. Then, from the head, through the bridge of the cervical spine, the shoulders redefine themselves on the ground. In this way, the position ceases to be a passive, propped-up position. The neck is freed as the arms come into play. Remember that Vanda never referred to Shoulderstand; instead she used the phrase neck-balance.
— Try using the shoulders in the same way in Uttanasana, Dog Pose and Handstand.

The Limbs

The function of arms and legs is always to relate to the spine. There are similarities, but also important differences, between the arms and the legs that we become aware of when we learn how to use them efficiently.

To discover how best to use the legs, first activate them to separate the two sides of the pelvis away from one another; then the feet and heels can open the knees. Now you can connect deeply into and through the legs before activating the spine.

Eventually, we can connect deeply through the legs, while releasing lightly through the arms. At first, this seems as difficult as rubbing the belly with one hand while patting the head with the other. As we refine our attention, it becomes easier.

The arms

The arms are the most elegant and finely jointed parts of the skeleton. They rest into the back torso before opening from the back of the spine. The arms are related not only to the muscles of the upper spine, but also to muscles deep in the pelvic basin. If this is forgotten, stiffness and pain often occur. If we learn to use the arms well, the shoulders function properly.

When using the arms, we often lose their connections with the lower part of the body, including the bottom of the spine. It seems to be harder to integrate the arms with the rest of the body than to integrate the legs.

The relationship between the shoulder joint, elbow and wrist can be more clearly understood if we use our imagination. We can compare our arms with the wings of a bird whose flying muscles come from the shoulders close to the body, and so bring our centre of gravity upwards.

We can also learn from bats, which swim through the air by folding their wings inward, lifting them while flying. This saves a great deal of energy. '*Bat wings represent evolution's re-purposing of a mammalian forelimb for flight*'.[20] It takes far more energy to lift an outstretched arm than one that is retracted.

It is interesting to explore the parts of the arm through the elbow, which functions as three joints in one. Its L-shape allows for elegance of movement. A better understanding of the function of this joint can help avoid many injuries — for example, carpal tunnel syndrome, tennis elbow, frozen shoulder and neck problems.

Vanda often showed us pictures of Egyptian figures in Backbend; the elbows were never braced or fully extended. Thus, the connection through the spine was not disturbed. With practice, the arms are able to extend freely without disturbing the rest of the body.

There is a rotational connection between the wrist and elbow joint and also between elbow joint and shoulder. These connections should not be lost, whatever position the arms are in. It is as if the shoulders and hands always look through the elbows.

Try this in Elbow Balance:

— Follow the pathway from the hands to the elbows and allow the lumbar spine to rest you towards the head. Now follow the pathway from the elbows towards the hands and allow the lumbar spine to connect to the very bottom of the spine.

— Now you can engage your forearms on the ground, and the shoulders become active and weight-bearing. The weight of the skull and forearms is dropping towards the ground. Your shoulders now hold the spine so they can rest you both downwards through the spine and up-wards through the spine, creating space in the shoulder joint.

— These two actions, that are at first separate, in time become harmonious.

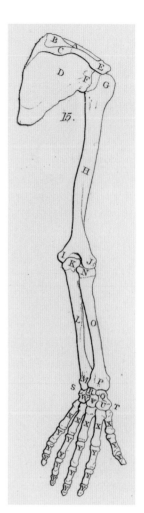

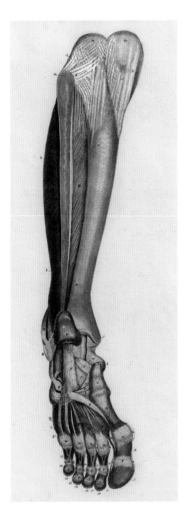

The legs

Locking our legs into position disturbs the dynamic connections through the legs and feet. We can learn how to use our legs better from cultures where walking barefoot and sitting on the ground are a way of life.

With intelligent use of the body, the legs can rediscover their lightness. Many of us may not have experienced this since we were infants.

Let's explore the leg below the knee joint. The fibula, or calf bone, is not part of the knee joint. It is part of the outer ankle, and can give elasticity and flexibility to the leg.

Vanda's instruction was to transfer weight to the outside of the feet. The ankles begin to rotate and the heels can then rest down.

The tibia, or shin bone, is the strongest weight-bearing bone in the body. Its upper end enters into the knee joint and its lower end is the talus, part of the ankle.

Vanda's instruction was, *'Gravitate properly on your heels with the knees straight.'* The knee sends weight down through the tibia and the heel transfers weight back upward through the tibia. Space is acquired in ankle and knee, allowing for their rotational freedom when the heel is engaged.

We often overwork our feet as if they were disconnected from the legs. Imagine your legs coming from within the pelvis. In this way, they can learn how to distribute weight to the feet. The feet need to have a chance to relax.

Later, when there is more understanding of the working of the foot in relation to the leg, the foot can become fully engaged. When the muscles in the soles of the feet learn to lengthen and contract more efficiently, leading to better cooperation between muscles and tendons, then we can feel more shifting and definition in the bones of the lower leg.

The Hands and Feet

The hands and feet contain half the bones in the body, so there are many potential connections to explore. Although they are similar in many ways, it is important to recognise their differences.

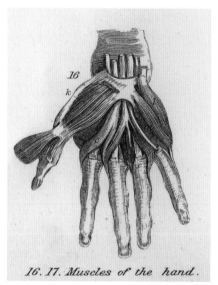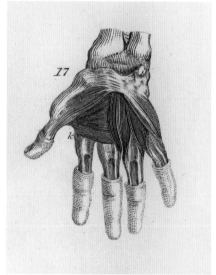

16. 17. Muscles of the hand.

The hands

The hands give accuracy to the way we use our arms. Be curious about the many diverse shapes and positions the hands can make. If we limit the hands' possibilities, it will make the shoulders and arms dull.

Like the foot, the hand has three arches. However, the thumb is unique — the only joint of its kind in the body. The thumb helps to keep space and rotation in the wrist, giving us more movement back and forth through the palm of the hand, which becomes a central axis.

Try this:

— Place your hand palm down, feed your thumb to the palm of the hand. Keeping the palm down, allow the hand to eat the thumb. Afterwards, the thumb frees itself and discovers a relationship both with the palm of the hand and with the wrist. This revitalises the 'spine' of the hand.

— Sit with your legs out in front of you. Use your hands as oars to row through imaginary water below. Sit on the outer pontoons of the legs so the hands and wrists are free to bring you upward through the spine.

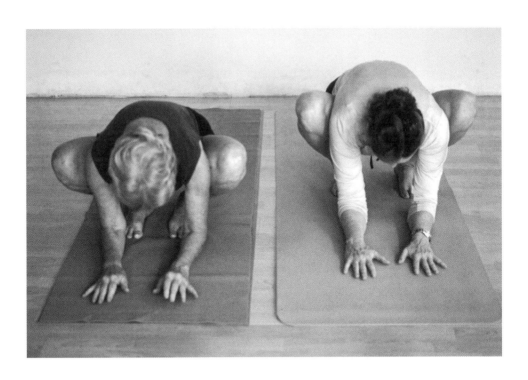

The feet

There are thirty-three joints and three arches in each foot, so there is unlimited possibility for discovering the rest of the body through the feet.

> 'The formation of the [longitudinal] arch in the foot, [both internal and external] is essential in order to stand and walk in a proper way. It can be obtained by directing the weight of the body on to the external part of the heel, keeping it down as long as possible while extending the sole towards the toes'.
>
> Vanda Scaravelli[21]

The front arch, in the ball of the foot, needs to be strengthened. It can then enliven the sole, whose tendons become the spine of the foot.

The foot works in a different way from the cupping action of the hands. The top of the foot becomes heavy, first to engage the sole of the foot from front to back, and then heavy again, to engage the sole of the foot from back to front. This keeps the ankles spacious and rotational, allowing weight to be distributed more efficiently throughout the legs. Only then can the heel be engaged.

It is best to think of the heel as separate from the rest of the foot. There's an important division between the cuboid bone of the middle of the foot and the

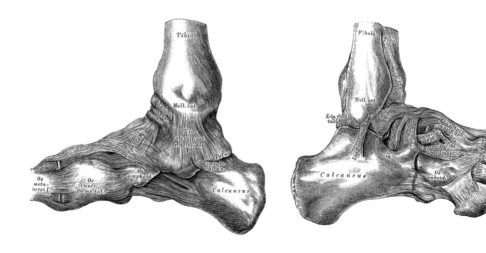

calcaneus talus. To find this division, the ankles must be made free and spacious, so that feet and lower leg muscles acquire more connections. This helps us lose the unhelpful habit of pressing down through the heel. Instead, we use the sole of the foot to deliver the heel down, without compression. Then, movement can be directed upward from the heels.

Experiment until you feel more space being invited in the ankle and femoral joint, helping to take tightness out of the thigh and calf muscles. We can regain natural movements that have been forgotten. The feet are designed to take the body's weight and, when working properly, they thrive on this.

> 'Tell your pupils to spread their "eyes", as much as possible, in the soles
> of their feet! It is incredibly important — and relaxes too'.
> Vanda Scaravelli in a letter to Sophy Hoare

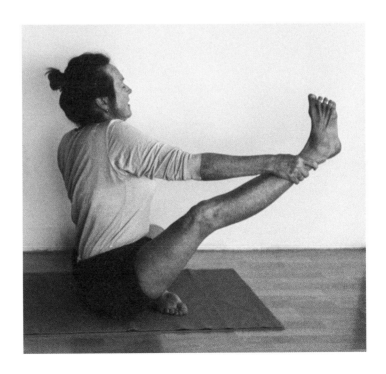

The Prominent Symphyses

Another way of looking at the body is to pay attention to the more prominent symphyses.

The skeleton of a newborn baby has around three hundred parts, which are predominantly composed of cartilage. An adult skeleton has two hundred and six parts. The cartilage is gradually replaced with bone, forming the adult skeleton. This growing together of the skeletal structure leaves us with some joints that are still entirely connected by cartilage. These are places where, at the beginning of our lives, we had much more freedom.

Nearly all the prominent symphyses lie in the central axis of the body: the joints between intervertebral discs, the sacro-coccygeal and pubic joints, the upper and lower joints in the sternum (the manubrium is the upper joint, and the xiphoid process is the lower), the jaw, and the joints of the skull. Much mobility can be regained as our body becomes more integrated.

As we become aware that the division in the spine is concentrated between the fourth and fifth lumbar vertebrae, the different segments of the spine come alive in interesting and new ways. Shoulder and thigh joints participate more fully in relation to the newly activated spine. They are designed to connect and work harmoniously together. We can relearn how to do this.

We can regain freedom behind and around the pubic symphysis, and in front of and around the sacro-coccygeal joint by bringing our centre of gravity upwards and engaging the outer thighs and heels. In time, this will enable us to find more space within the symphyses of the upper and lower sternum. The muscles at the base of the pelvis will become more responsive for participation in breathing.

The strong joint of the jaw consists of two broad vertical bones in front of the ears joined at the symphysis of the mandible. The face is made up of fourteen bones — so much opportunity to lose or gain a bit of space! When there is more space in the jaw, more space is created between the bones of the face.

The jaw muscles can easily become clenched, creating tension in the neck and the top of the spine. As we learn to free the spine, little by little, this tension eases.

The joints remember an earlier freedom. The spinal fluid is no longer obstructed and is able to flow freely up and down the spine.

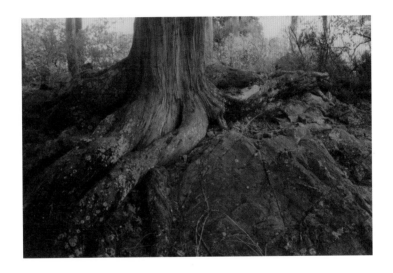

'You have to understand the form of the body in order to understand the meaning of light from within it.'

Jalaluddin Rumi[22]

Through play and imagination, we gradually expand our understanding of anatomy. When our mode becomes more playful, we begin to find out how to move. Our observations and spontaneous wonderings incite a more piercing scientific enquiry. Play leads to real insights that offer up meaningful discoveries.

Breathing

'Nerves and muscles of the three systems — breathing, speech and locomotion — must interact.... And so we find that the structure of the mechanism for speech and breathing serves also, in its cartilaginous, ligamentous, bony and muscular traction, as a part of the tensile posture mechanism of the entire body.'

Mabel E. Todd[23]

Fig. 3.

LUNGS OF A BIRD.

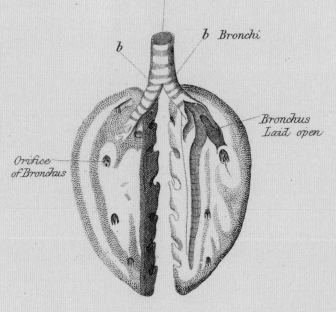

a Trachea

b Bronchi

b

*Bronchus
Laid open*

*Orifice
of Bronchus*

Natural Rhythms

Breathing and locomotion developed together when we became land creatures. How we use our arms, legs, feet, hips and shoulders affects the way we breathe, as well as the way we move. Lungs and diaphragm are parts of the body's whole dynamic structure.

It is unhelpful to control the breath directly during asana practice, although many schools of yoga recommend it (for example, exhaling on bending forward and inhaling on standing upright again, or forcefully exhaling on every movement). This interferes with the body's natural drive towards integration. Trust that the breath will come and go in its own rhythm.

After practising for a few years, centring on the spine, you will notice that your breathing starts to change, sometimes in unexpected ways. It acquires a more spontaneous, natural movement which arises from the conditions you have created through attentive practice.

As we work at raising our centre of gravity by moving upwards through the spine, our lungs acquire more space. The action of the diaphragm no longer pushes the belly out and we can stop holding the rib-cage. We become less tense, quieter on the surface, as we take our attention within, towards the spine and lungs. We free the living creature inside the shell!

For many of us, the more difficult part of our practice to establish is Pranayama. It takes some years to develop a relationship with the lungs. Yoga books and classes often emphasise the role of the diaphragm with little reference to the lungs. Vanda used to place a picture of the lungs beside us while we were practising Pranayama with her. She would keep our attention focused on the depth, rhythm, and pleasure of the breath. In time, the back of the skull and the base of the spine were involved in perceiving the lungs and the tasks they were performing. How much more space could be given to them! This alert participation with the breath began to change the musculature which, in turn, led to a better understanding of the asanas.

It is estimated that we participate in seventeen to twenty thousand breaths per day — between eight and twenty breaths a minute. The lungs have a capacity of about six litres, of which only a very small amount is normally used — maybe half a litre. We tend to concentrate our breathing in the upper part of the lungs. Yet, the largest number of air sacs is in the lower section.

Learning to breathe more efficiently, we revitalise our bodies, making better use of the incoming oxygen and expelling carbon dioxide more effectively.

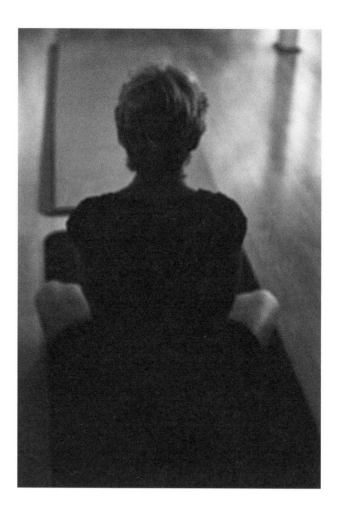

Sitting

Students in yoga classes are often taught to sit on the floor and bring regularity to inhalation and exhalation, with little attention paid to achieving a relaxed and alert position. Collapse occurs, followed by the fight against collapse, which creates tension in the back muscles. Sometimes breathing is taught too forcefully, causing tension around the upper and lower spine.

The 'sitting bones' are not our base for sitting. Instead, there is a transfer of weight from thighs to lumbar spine through the hips; the feet and lower legs are then engaged. The knees acquire more space. The position should be able to renew itself and not become uncomfortable.

Exploring how to sit from standing, and how to stand from sitting, can help us become more comfortable when seated.

Notice how shallow breathing interferes with the movement of the arms, creates tension in the neck and pulls the weight of the shoulders onto the ribcage so that the clavicle is constrained. The weight of the body should not sink, but should be redirected upwards.

The lower body, below the lungs, is involved in helping the lungs fill upwards.

The top of the body, above the lungs, is lightened — shoulders free, arms light, head and neck letting go of their holding.

In the middle of the body, closer to the lungs, from the top of the pelvis to the skull, there is interplay between the thoracic and lumbar vertebrae.

Fig. 2.

HUMAN CHEST.

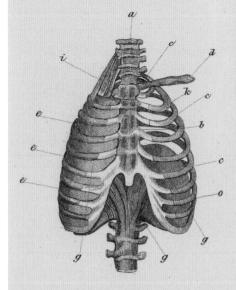

a. Backbone (neck)
b. Breastbone.
c.c. Ribs.
d. Clavicle.
e. Inter-costal muscles.
g. Diaphragm.
i. Muscles of the neck.

Fig. 1.

HUMAN LUNGS.

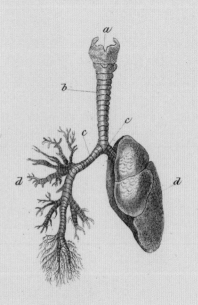

a. larynx.
b. windpipe.
c.c. bronchi.
d. bronchial tubes.

Visualising the Breath

Instead of the commonly used analogy of a balloon, Vanda often used a sponge to show how the lungs work. She would squeeze a damp sponge from bottom to top, leaving it empty and light, ready to absorb again. She also gave us a broomstick to place under our armpits, with our arms resting over it, so head and shoulders could re-arrange themselves for lighter, freer breathing. It is important to use our imagination, especially when we come to breathing. Each image we become engaged with and enter into will bring a certain understanding, which will then free us to begin again with a new image.

We can imagine we are like birds, which have a very efficient respiratory system for flying, often at altitudes, where oxygen is scarce. Their lung capacity is augmented by air sacs inside their bones and body cavities. Air passes through their lungs, like water through a sponge, in a constant circulatory movement so that, unlike mammals, the lungs never deflate.

We don't have air sacs, but we can engage our lower limbs in such a way that our centre of gravity is raised and we become lighter. The horizontal division of the spine's centre is shifted upwards through the centre of the lungs, as if to help us fly.

When we sit and watch the breath, we can experience a bird-like lightness and a softly circular rhythm.

Inhalation

Phase 1

Do: You need do nothing except collect outer thighs and hips towards the spine.

Observe: As your feet and the base of your spine drop, the breath spreads and expands into the lower section of the lungs.

Phase 2

Do: You need do nothing except lighten your shoulders.

Observe: The hips accompany the breath as it spreads out within the middle section of the lungs.

Phase 3:

Do: You need do nothing except lighten and empty your arms, keeping your head free above the spine.

Observe: The breath enters spontaneously into the upper section of the lungs. Now, there can be a moment of rest and ease before the beginning of the exhalation.

Exhalation

Phase 1:

Observe: In the wide, full, upper body, the breath begins to be released out through the lungs.

Phase 2:

Engage: Return to the spine so that the deeper muscles along the spine can send the breath out of the lungs.

There is an old story from the Middle East, used here as a metaphor for the role of the breath as a link between body and mind.

The King's Escape

Once upon a time, there was a king who had a wise and loyal minister. His commander-in-chief plotted against the king and imprisoned him in a room at the top of a tall tower. The room had a window which opened, but it was too high to escape from. The minister conceived a plan. He captured a honey bee and fixed a small stick on to its head, then applied a drop of honey to the other end of the stick. He let the bee go at the bottom of the tower, where the bee smelt the honey above and flew up to find it.

The minister had tied a fine silken thread to the body of the bee. As it rose past the window, the king caught hold of it. Then, the minister tied a thick cotton thread to the other end of the silken one. The king pulled it up until he could catch hold of the cotton thread. The minister tied a thick rope to his end of the cotton thread and, as before, the king pulled it up into his room. He knotted the rope, secured it and climbed down to the ground.

The Simple Breath

We can use the voice to free the breath. Vanda used the 'ha!' sound. Buzzing, deep humming and hissing can also be helpful; the breath can ride freely on the wave of sound.

The exhalation is potentially about one and a half times longer than the in-breath. Imagine that the exhalation has two phases, the first from within the lungs upwards, as if from the centre of the spine, lightly through the nostrils. Then there is a freer, deeper release upwards through the throat and nostrils; you may notice a horizontal expansion through shoulders and hips.

In this way, the lower part of the lungs, where the most significant gas exchange takes place, regains elasticity. As in asana practice, we eventually discover the vital area of the fourth-fifth lumbar, enabling the coccyx to unfurl away from the sacrum. It goes further away from, and also finds its connection to, the base of the skull. An old memory is awakened and we begin to find more space at the top and bottom of the sternum and between the bones of the skull and jaw.

At the end of the exhalation there is a slight pause, as if the breath learns from the heart and diaphragm that the rest period is longer than the working phase. You will feel how this allows the adjoining musculature to become more toned. Mabel Todd, in *The Thinking Body,*[24] describes it as, *'re-establishing the potential energy balance before allowing it to be employed again.'*

Then, the inhalation comes and the lungs begin filling from the deep back — slowly — so the rest of the body rearranges itself to let this happen — receiving, not taking. If we don't interfere, the diaphragm can expand and contract fully, keeping the belly relaxed and reducing the work of the heart.

There can be an interesting play between the involvement of the lower body and the quality of ease in the upper body. Be present, and let progress happen bit by bit. Beware of habit and be attentive to rhythm. Perhaps, thinking of the lungs as divided into three sections — lower, middle and upper — can enhance the rhythmical quality of the breath.

Beginning Your Pranayama Practice

The images we suggest here are a launching pad towards a richer understanding of breathing and are not to be held on to. You can begin by sitting for five minutes at a time. Don't endure discomfort — let yourself be drawn to stay with stillness. If necessary, change your position to ease an area of tension, so that you can continue to observe the lungs without distraction. You do not need to impose timing on the breath. Vanda suggested touching the pulse in one wrist to follow its rhythm for inhalation and exhalation.

Comfort, rest, rhythm — these three qualities can encourage you to spend longer periods watching and participating in the work of the lungs. Take your time; be generous in preparing for the breath — more spacious, emptier. Just as Vanda warmly welcomed many guests from all over the world and entertained them, she encouraged us in this way to approach the breath. In time, you can relax your

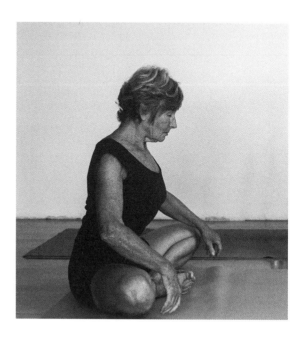

focus on the changing conditions within the lungs and broaden the scope of your attention, refining it, so that it can encompass more than one thing at a time. You begin to notice the unexpected. Each part of the body can renew itself as it accommodates the breath.

Variations on Breathing

You can use the following exercises to help refine your simple Pranayama practice. When you become familiar with them, you can move on and create your own exercises, finding rhythm and imagery to keep the practice fresh and absorbing.

Kapalabhati:

This exercise involves a series of short expulsions of breath through the nostrils. It is important not to pull inwards with the belly, forcing the abdominal muscles. Avoid tightening the buttocks. Do not push the air out of the nostrils, but exhale as if from the back of the skull.

Try freeing the shoulders and hips so you feel the breath lightened upwards through the lungs. Remember to engage your thighs with the ground, using your feet to give you a sense of sitting through your legs, as if keeping the option to stand up. There should be a lessening of tension in the groins, sacrum and around the anus.

Retention of breath (Viloma):

During exhalation, after receiving the breath, let it go gradually, a little at a time, like a curtain at a window which is lifted by the breeze and dropped again a few times before coming to rest.

During inhalation, let the lungs fill a little, then savour the pause. Inhale a little more, becoming engaged with the pause — and so on, three or four times, so that the pause itself becomes a vital part of the dance.

'Breathing is the most important part of yoga practice. Once we start breathing, training cannot be interrupted, it must be done regularly each day.'

Vanda Scaravelli[25]

Teaching

'*…sometimes it is necessary to re-teach a thing its loveliness…*'

Galway Kinnell [26]

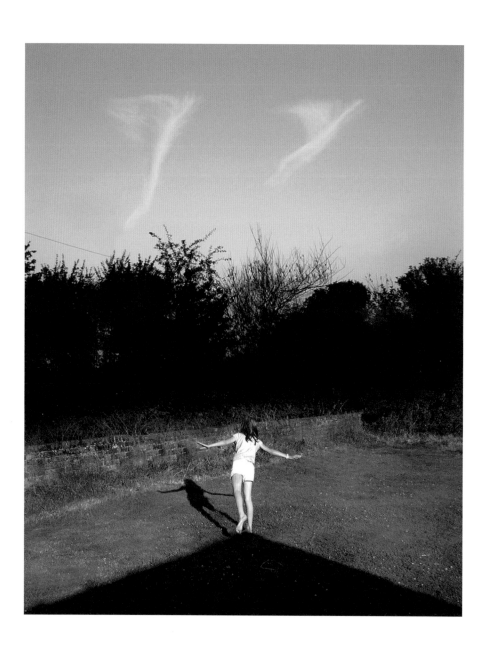

Reflections

The way that this practice demands to be taught, and the way that Vanda taught, has similarities with some of the esoteric teachings, such as the hermetic tradition, alchemy and Zen. At first, students can feel disorientated because the new cannot be defined in terms of the old. It is up to the students to use their imagination, and to tolerate not knowing. It is an intimate and personal process.

The practice, and the teaching of it, can be full of contradictions, often mystifying, but enlightening when the paradox is understood. The student has to have a taste for this kind of learning and a strong desire to discover what it leads to. Otherwise, the process will be impossible to embrace.

Sophy

At the end of a lesson, Vanda would invite me to lie on my back and relax with a soft beanbag over my eyes. To my slight annoyance Vanda would throw the bag carelessly in such a way that it always seem to land more heavily on my left eye than on my right. One day, in another context, I explained to Vanda that my head had a tendency to roll towards the right, where upon she replied, *'that is why I give more weight to the left when you are resting.'*

Sometimes we become frustrated in our efforts to deepen our practice; it takes time to learn from our teachers and to gain the understanding of our own bodies' intelligence. We can trust the state of not knowing because it is the source of our discoveries. Learning often takes place in ways that surprise us.

> *'It's not only a matter of the disciple grasping the truth of what he is told. The teacher also needs to catch something, and keep catching it. He doesn't have some fixed knowledge, but needs to discover it freshly at every moment. [...] The truth flows so rapidly that anything you think you know is not the truth, because knowing is too slow.'*
>
> Peter Kingsley[27]

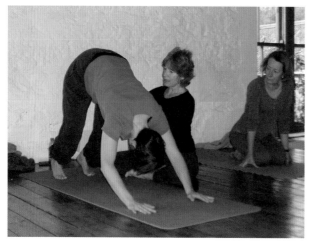

This demands a subtle alertness. Our attention must be focused and totally present.

Our teaching springs from our own practice; when something becomes clear in our own bodies, there is no analysis, only attention. From our practice, we can see and feel into another's body and guide them intuitively.

When we teach, we are putting trust in our experience rather than in rules. Our students trust us because they sense the authenticity of our knowledge, and they can observe us demonstrating everything we say. They will understand that they are engaged in a process, which will keep evolving as long as they continue to practise. And, those who have developed a regular practice often have to start teaching themselves, not only to pass on the beautiful practice to others, but also because one learns so much by doing so.

Vanda was always learning from herself as she taught. Her fascination with the steps of learning was transmitted to her students. How much less? How much further? What could and could not be altered?

Diane

Vanda's hands were teaching me to integrate my knees into asanas. After taking several months of Tai Chi lessons together, this all changed. At times, my lessons would begin with 'What do you want to do today?' I would respond; she would do something completely different. Years later, she began walking daily by the country road, leading with her penetrating heels, palms together behind her back. This is when she taught me to use the arms as wings and become a bird, no longer a woman. In the last years of her life, as her piano playing acquired a different intensity, so too did her teaching of the breath. There was no usual lesson with Vanda.

For us, teaching is about helping students to explore asanas, discovering pathways and connections throughout the body. Experienced 'hands on' teaching is important for helping the body respond to these new connections. However, our attention is repeatedly brought back to the whole body, even when focusing on one area.

Relating postures to each other, rather than seeing them as distinct entities, allows us to devise our own sequences. Surprise yourself with the ways you combine postures; Sun Salutation was once invented by someone experimenting. After first exploring the most relaxed part of our body in one practice, we can change in a subsequent practice and start with the least relaxed part. It is only through playfulness that the beginner's mind may be uncovered. Vanda often said, *'Be like a child.'* When we teach, we have to cast around for new ways of saying things, keeping our attention fresh. We need to use a round about way of thinking.

Sometimes 'adjusting' can interfere with a deeper understanding of the body, for both teacher and student. Learn to use the brain like a pair of hands to hold, direct, and accompany movement. In time, hands acquire a new intelligence.

In one of my favourite moments with Vanda, the telephone rang during a lesson. A violinist needed help with an upcoming concert.

With the receiver held between her head and shoulder, and gesticulating with one hand, she gave verbal instructions to the violinist while helping me with her other hand and foot. She made it all seem simple and natural.

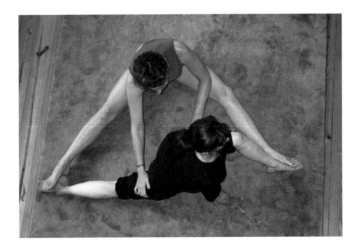

Vanda Scaravelli the Teacher

The following article was written by our friend, Elizabeth Pauncz, in February 2000. It evokes, so vividly, our own experience of Vanda that we wanted to reproduce excerpts from it here. Elizabeth has kindly given us permission to include it.

Vanda began teaching very late in life. In fact, her modesty was such that, when asked to teach, she would say, *'there is nothing to teach'* which, with most things, was only a partial truth. Her special gift for understanding yoga was truly remarkable and she shared this with anyone in immeasurable generosity. She was not particularly fond of talking but rather acted spontaneously and with supreme confidence.

She thought very carefully and at length before accepting a student, often postponing or refusing him or her, so great was her commitment to the responsibility and importance of yoga.

Part of the brilliance of Vanda's teaching lay in the fact that she gave very few instructions, always saying that the body has to learn to 'undo' and 'let go', which is not a state of passivity but alert watchfulness so it can find its natural way of existing. Her approach to yoga followed this same line of thought: rigor, precision and clarity through total attention to what was happening in the precise moment. She lived in the present moment, rarely talking about either the past or of the future.

'Past is past,' she would say from time to time when questioned.

She taught each person individually in the bedroom of her house in the Tuscan countryside. No day was the same, although she would repeat the same instructions over and over. Each time they carried a new meaning and brought new levels of understanding such was the depth of her knowledge.

Sometimes she would throw a photocopy of the lungs at my feet before we practised breathing and it would stay there for the entire lesson. The same photocopy would appear twenty more times and once in a while my mind would object, thinking, 'but I've seen this', only to realize immediately that I had not really grasped the meaning yet and that there was always more to understand.

Other days we would study photographs and then proceed with a position. We examined Krishnamacharya with a magnifying glass many times. We studied how birds used their feet in taking off into flight or landing and then practised that same technique in Tadasana, which would lead to Urdhva Dhanurasana. We usually did the positions together; sometimes she would go first and illustrate a certain point.

Another way she taught was through touch and sensation. I would put my hands on a particular area of her body to feel how it moved and reacted and then try to imitate this.

She cut through all details. 'There is so much joy in teaching what you feel is right. This changed perception will give you wings to find the best words and adequate expressions to transmit what you have seen with your mind.'

All the incongruities of life could be present in a lesson. I came to accept them and allow myself to open up into a larger dimension where all events helped my practice and led me to greater concentration, teaching me how to return again and again to an asana, each time drawing a little closer to understanding. Through practice and attention movements 'unfolded' by themselves, creating space for enjoyment.

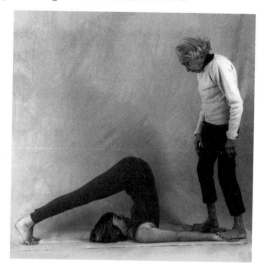

'You must learn something new each time you do yoga.' It was not a repetition, rather a new experience each time we began. 'Teaching starts with freedom and ends with freedom.'

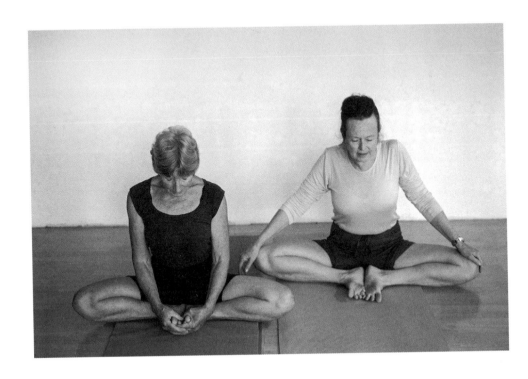

Diane

After I had been studying with Vanda for several years, she insisted I go to teach a group of 'advanced teachers' in the United States. I tried my best to convince her otherwise. Trying to convince Vanda did not usually work, and it didn't on this occasion. After returning from my trip, I was surprised that Vanda didn't ask me about the experience. Shyly, I began the conversation, *'Vanda, you know I taught the group of teachers in the United States.'* She did not respond. I repeated myself, thinking she hadn't heard me, adding, *'It was difficult for me.'* She finished whatever she was doing, probably brushing her hair or peeling garlic cloves, walked over to me, took my wrist, looked at me briefly and said, *'It's not about you.'*

Sophy

During the time I worked with Vanda, I dreamt that she came to visit me. We were in a large rectangular room with windows all down one side overlooking a garden, with light streaming through them.

There was a grand piano at one end and a fireplace at the other. The top of the piano was completely covered with plants.

As the dream went on, Vanda started looking younger and younger. She was exactly as I remember her in life, but her face was now very young and free of lines, and instead of wearing her usual yoga clothes she wore a more conventional, elegant outfit — her 'going away' clothes.

Then she gave me a big fond embrace and said, *'Sophy, I won't see you again'*. I didn't know if she meant it literally — part of me wanted to protest: *'But we haven't even done any yoga!'* Then, she went out through the front door of the house and I followed her. There was a cortège of smart black cars, like a funeral, waiting for her and I was aware that members of her family were there. She got into one of the cars, but when I ran up to it to look in, she had vanished. In the car was a newborn baby lying in a basket.

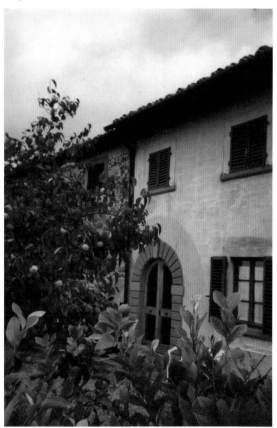

The principles of yoga can be shared and transmitted. Vanda would sometimes quote Iyengar, who used the phrase, 'Now you can go, any amount,' referring to the fact that the conditions were right and everything had been attended to. While the qualities and challenges of this yoga offer pleasure to the body and implore the imagination to participate, the subtleties reveal themselves only through time and practice. The individual expression of this process is always unique and in a state of becoming.

'On the way to knowledge
Many things are accumulated.
On the way to wisdom
Many things are discarded.
Less and less effort is used
Until things arrange themselves.'

Lao Tzu[28]

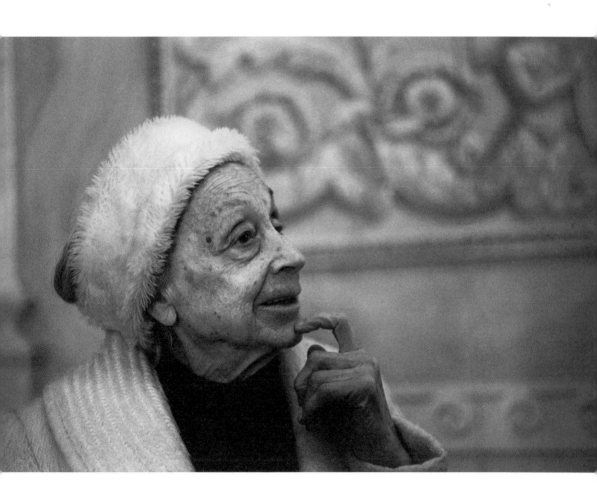

with gratitude, Diane and Sophy

Acknowledgements

We would, first and foremost, like to thank Annette Heyer and Lise Bratton for their editorial and design work, which has transformed our words into this beautiful book.

Diane

I personally would like to acknowledge and express my gratitude to all the students who are the muses of my practice of yoga. You are too many to name, but thank you for your curiosity, your interest, your devotion, your disagreement and your growing discernment.

And thank you to my wonderful sons, Angus and Taillefer, who have put up with a yoga mom for as long as they can remember.

Sophy

I wish to thank Annette for the all the time and trouble she has taken helping me complete my work on the book

And to thank Sasha, my daughter, and Pete, my partner, for the work they have done on the book, and for their encouragement and support throughout the process of bringing this book to fruition.

Illustrations

The publisher, authors and editors wish to thank the following for allowing the reproduction of their photographs and illustrations:

Alexandra Gray   p. 125: *Diane Teaching*, Blowing Rock, N. Carolina, courtesy Diane Long

Alexandra Sotiropoulou   p. 50: *Egyptian Relief Sculpture*, National Archaeological Museum Collection, Athens

Annette Heyer   pp. 10, 11, 12, 23, 26, 27, 34, 35, 38, 43, 55, 66, 67, 68, 69, 72, 73, 75, 86, 88, 89, 90, 91, 94, 95, 96, 97, 103, 105, 112, 118, 128: *Diane and Sophy Practising, London, September 2014,* courtesy Annette Heyer, copyright A.Heyer

Collection Annette Heyer   Anatomical Etchings:
p. 100: *Arm and shoulder*
p. 101: *Muscles and Tendons of the Lower Leg and Foot*
p. 102: *Muscles of the Hand*
p. 110: *Bird Lung*
p. 114: *Human Lung*

Arthuro Patten   p. 127: *Vanda Teaching*, courtesy of Elisabeth Pauncz

Ben Gold   p. 40: *Snowy Trees*, courtesy Sophy Hoare, copyright B. Gold

Bernhard Siegfried Albinus   pp. 42, 80: from *Tables of the Skeleton and Muscles, 1749,* Wellcome Images, London, under Creative Commons licence CC BY 4.0

Diane Long   p. 16: *Vanda Unlocking the Door*
p. 129: *Vanda's House*
p. 107: *Vanda's Favourite Tree*
p. 41: *Diane in Tree House*
p. 13: *Diane Practising*
p. 30: *Neume*, with kind permission of the Library at Farfa Abbey, Northern Lazio, Italy

Glossary of Poses

Below are the poses illustrated, with their English and Sanskrit names.

References

Introduction

1. Vanda Scaravelli, *Awakening the Spine,* Pinter & Martin, London, 2012

Becoming a Beginner

2. Wendell Berry, *The Real Work* in *Standing by Words,* Counterpoint Press, Berkley,1983
3. Mabel E. Todd, *The Thinking Body,* Dance Horizons (Princeton Book Company), Princeton, 1937

The Quality of Practice

4. Rabindranath Tagore, *Steam of Life LXIX, Gitanjali, Song Offerings,* McMillen & Co., London, 1913
5. Plato, *The Republic,* Penguin Classics, London, 2007
6. Novalis (Friederich von Hardenberg), see Oliver Sachs, *Musicophilia: Tales of Music and the Brain,* Vintage Books (Knopf Doubleday), 2008
7. Nicephorus the Solitary, *The Prayer of the Heart,* adapted from writings in *The Philokalia,* translated by E. Kadloubosky and G.E.H. Palmer, Faber & Faber, London, 1992
8. Rainer Maria Rilke, *The Complete French Poems;* translated by A. Poulin, Jr., Graywolf Press, 2002
9. Michael M. Merzenich, Professor Emeritus Neuroscientist at the University of California, San Francisco; see *Growing Evidence of Brain Plasticity* | TED Talk, www.ted.com/talks/michael_merzenich_on_the_elastic_brain?language=en
10. Mark Solms and Oliver Turnbull, *The Brain and the Inner World: An Introduction to the Neuroscience of Subjective Experience,* Other Press, New York, 2002
11. For an explanation of F. M. Alexander and the Alexander Technique, see www.alexandertechnique.com/fma.htm
12. Solms & Turnbull, ibid.

Elegant Architecture

13. Mabel E. Todd, ibid.

14. Leonardo da Vinci, *The Notebooks of Leonardo da Vinci*, (*XIII Theoretical Writings on Architecture*); ed. Jean Paul Richter in 1880; Dover, 1970

15. Wendell Berry, *The Gift of Gravity*, in *New Collected Poems*; Counterpoint Press; Berkeley, 2012

Questionning Asana

16. Sri Anandamayi, reproduced with the kind permission of the Ma Anandamayi Foundation

17. Attributed to the Song Dynasty Daoist Priest Zhang Sanfeng, *Tai Ji Quan Treatise*, Stuart Alve Olson, Createspace, January 2011

Rethinking Anatomy

18. Vanda Scaravelli, ibid.

19. Vanda Scaravelli, ibid.

20. See www.wired.com/2012/04/bat-wings-flight/. Also *Upstroke Wing Flexion and the Inertial Cost of Bat Flight*, Daniel K. Riskin, Attila Bergou, Kenneth S. Breurer and Sharon M. Swartz; Proceedings of the Royal Society B, 2012

21. Vanda Scaravelli, ibid.

22. See *The Rumi Collection, An Anthology of Translations of Mevlana Jalaluddin Rumi*; Shambhala Publications Inc, 2005

Breathing

23. Mabel E. Todd, ibid.

24   Mabel E. Todd, ibid.

25. Vanda Scaravelli, ibid.

Teaching

26. Galway Kinnell, *Saint Francis and the Sow* in *A New Selected Poems*, First Mariner Books (Houghton Mifflin Company), Boston, 2001

27. Peter Kingsley, *Knowing Beyond Knowing*, Parabola Vol. XXII/1, 1997

28. Lao Tzu, *The Complete Works of Lao Tzu: Tao Teh Ching and Hua Hu Ching*, Sevenstar Communications, 1993

Notes

Notes

Notes